Handbook of Integrated Short–Term Psychotherapy

Handbook of Integrated Short-Term Psychotherapy

Arnold Winston, M.D.

*Chairman, Department of Psychiatry,
Beth Israel Medical Center
Professor and Vice Chairman, Department of Psychiatry,
Albert Einstein College of Medicine
New York, New York*

Beverly Winston, Ph.D.

*Supervising Psychotherapist, Department of Psychiatry,
Beth Israel Medical Center
Assistant Clinical Professor of Psychiatry,
Albert Einstein College of Medicine
Faculty, New York School for
Psychoanalytic Psychotherapy and Psychoanalysis
New York, New York*

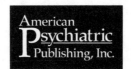

American Psychiatric Publishing, Inc.

Washington, DC
London, England

Copyright © 2002 American Psychiatric Publishing, Inc.

05 04 03 02   4 3 2 1

ALL RIGHTS RESERVED

Manufactured in the United States of America on acid-free paper

American Psychiatric Publishing, Inc.
1400 K Street, NW
Washington, DC 20005
www.appi.org

Library of Congress Cataloging-in-Publication Data
Winston, Arnold, 1935– .
    Handbook of integrated short-term psychotherapy / Arnold Winston, Beverly Winston.
        p. ; cm.
    Includes bibliographical references and index.
    ISBN 0-88048-814-X (alk. paper)
    1. Brief psychotherapy. I. Winston, Beverly, 1938– . II. Title.
    [DNLM: 1. Psychotherapy, Brief—methods. WM 420.5.P5 W783h 2001]
    RC480.55 W56 2001
    616.89′14—dc21
                                                                2001022960

British Library Cataloguing in Publication Data

A CIP record is available from the British Library.

To our patients, from whom we have learned so much;
to our students, who have challenged us to explain what we have learned;
to our children, Roy, Eric and Jane, Michael and Jill;
and to our grandchildren, Emma and Joshua.

Contents

CHAPTER

1

CHAPTER

2

CHAPTER

3

Assessment and Case Formulation 23

CHAPTER

4

The Therapeutic Relationship 57

CHAPTER

5

Essential Elements and Interventions............73

CHAPTER

6

The Partnership:
Medication and Psychotherapy......................95

CHAPTER

7

Initial Phase of Treatment 107

CHAPTER

8

CHAPTER

9

CHAPTER
10

Preface

The motivation for writing this book comes from our experience in teaching brief integrated psychotherapy to mental health professionals and students. We have found that students as well as experienced clinicians have difficulty conceptualizing and using an integrated, multimodal approach. Most psychotherapists are trained in only one model of psychotherapy; however, many patients are better served by a treatment model that incorporates many different types of interventions. Too often, patients are asked to fit into a particular psychotherapy without consideration of the possibility that it may not be the appropriate approach for them. We believe that an integrated approach offers the opportunity to apply therapeutic interventions differentially, enabling the therapist to tailor treatment to the patient.

In the past, the efficacy of brief treatment was relatively unknown, and brief treatment was practiced by few clinicians. Today, many therapists are using time-limited approaches because of patient preference and external pressure from insurance companies. However, some clinicians still entertain the belief that brief treatments are inferior or stopgap at best. Research evidence indicates otherwise: although extended, open-ended approaches are best for certain chronic, debilitating illnesses, short-term treatment can be as efficacious as long-term therapy for many disorders and problems.

In this book we outline a system of therapeutics with differential application according to patient assessment, diagnosis, and case formulation. We describe an integrated brief psychotherapy approach based on this system that incorporates cognitive-behavioral, interpersonal, and psychoanalytically derived expressive and supportive treatments.

Four major areas are addressed within this framework:

1. Understanding, conceptualizing, and formulating patients' problems
2. Setting realistic treatment goals
3. Knowing what to say to patients (technique)
4. Maintaining a positive therapeutic alliance

In addition to these four areas, we discuss the important issue of medication and its integration with psychotherapy, as well as significant research findings regarding combined treatment.

An understanding of patients' problems is essential in conducting all psychotherapy, but especially brief psychotherapy. Traditionally, therapists have been taught to allow patient material to unfold. In brief psychotherapy, a concise formulation must be developed within the first few hours of treatment so that the therapist can understand and focus on the patient's core problems early in therapy. We describe a detailed method of patient assessment and case formulation as the cornerstone of our model of short-term treatment.

The first building block in conducting brief treatment is establishing goals with the patient. In traditional long-term therapy, goals are often left undefined, with some implicit idea that problems, when talked about and understood, will be resolved. In brief treatment, goals are made explicit from the beginning. They are derived from the patient's desire for change and the therapist's understanding of what is possible for the patient. Setting realistic goals depends on completing a careful evaluation; listening to the patient's wishes, desires, and dissatisfactions; and establishing agreement about what the work of therapy will encompass.

All practitioners search for more effective ways to approach patients, and we believe that the student or clinician attempting to practice brief treatment needs clear guidelines for the conduct and progression of psychotherapy from beginning to end. Such guidelines must provide focused, concrete techniques as opposed to more general approaches. There is great diversity of theoretical and technical approaches to brief psychotherapy as practiced by a number of pioneers in the field (Beck, Davanloo, Ellis, Malan, Mann, Sifneos, and others). Clinicians and students have noted that even after reviewing and understanding the considerable literature on technique in brief treatment, they often have difficulty applying the specific treatments and knowing what to say to patients. Although we discuss each of these different points of view, we emphasize a more unified treatment that integrates the various approaches. This integration is based on the evaluation and case formulation. We stress the differential use of therapeutic interventions, employing the continuum of interpretative to supportive approaches (including cognitive-behavioral and interpersonal techniques). Case examples of patients with different types of problems and psychopathology are presented to illustrate the use of these techniques.

The importance of the therapeutic alliance has been well documented. Psychotherapy research has clearly demonstrated that the quality of the therapeutic alliance is the best predictor of outcome in psychotherapy. In brief psychotherapy, it is vital to maintain the alliance and to quickly repair any breaches that occur. We present a framework for preserving and enhancing the alliance and for remedying misunderstandings between patient and therapist.

Although the integration of psychotherapy and pharmacotherapy has been fraught with difficulties, most clinicians recognize the need for such integration and use a combined approach in their work with patients. In what follows, a model is presented for a collaborative approach, as well as a summary of the past 20 years of research findings on combined treatment.

Historically, there have been some controversies regarding the efficacy of short-term treatment and its power to achieve lasting change. We review the literature, presenting evidence from current research studies that should help clinicians feel confident in the power of brief treatment. Despite major advances in psychotherapy outcome and process research, practitioners have been largely unaware of important findings that can serve as powerful guides to the practice of brief treatment.

Acknowledgments

We are indebted to a number of friends and colleagues for their help during the writing of this book. Stuart Feder encouraged us to put pen to paper, was our sounding board, provided a helpful review of each chapter, and gave us his time and wisdom. Christopher Muran provided important feedback on cognitive-behavioral therapy and its relationship to other approaches. Harold Been made useful suggestions for the evaluation and theory chapters. We would like to thank our editor from American Psychiatric Publishing, Inc., Rebecca Richters, for editing our manuscript with thoroughness and sensitivity.

We are grateful to the pioneers in the field of brief psychotherapy who influenced our thinking—in particular, Habib Davanloo, David Malan, and Peter Sifneos, for the foundation for our work, and Aaron Beck, for the cognitive-behavioral component of our approach.

Finally, we wish to acknowledge the importance of the Beth Israel Psychotherapy Research Program in providing the impetus for this book, and our colleagues from this program, especially Christopher Muran, Jeremy Safran, Lisa Wallner Samstag, Michael Laiken, Henry Pinsker, Richard Rosenthal, Lee McCullough, and Manuel Trujillo.

Arnold Winston, M.D.
Beverly Winston, Ph.D.

CHAPTER

1

History of
Brief Psychotherapy

This book is a guide for clinicians and advanced students practicing brief treatment. We present an integrated approach for patient evaluation, case formulation, and treatment to enable clinicians to practice with clear guidelines. At the same time, we highlight the importance of the patient-therapist relationship, according special attention to its centrality in brief treatment.

Introduction

There has always been an interest in shortening psychotherapy (Ferenczi and Rank 1925/1956), and in the past few years, brief treatment has flourished for a number of reasons. First, more and more therapists have become interested in the practice of brief treatment, recognizing that for many individuals it can and does accomplish as much as long-term treatment. As a result, brief treatment has thrived and, indeed, is the treatment of choice for many patients.

Second, the acceptance of more limited goals by mental health professionals has aided the growth of brief treatment. There have always been patients whose aim is symptom relief, help with one specific area in their lives

1

or personality functioning, or improvement in their relationship with a child, partner, parent, or boss. For this population, brief treatment is a natural choice.

Third, a number of individuals who enter therapy already have an understanding of their problems, which are often circumscribed. In addition, their motivation to work hard in treatment makes them good candidates for brief psychotherapy.

Fourth, many individuals have financial constraints, limited time, and little interest in sustaining a long-term treatment. They think about and use psychotherapy in much the same way as they think about and use primary care medicine. Their desire is to be treated in a timely fashion with rapid resolution of their problems.

Fifth, approaches such as crisis intervention and cognitive-behavioral therapy have always been effective methods for delivering services to many people in a time-limited fashion. The crisis intervention approach has influenced the field in the direction of briefer treatments for people who have been through disasters or severe trauma.

Sixth, managed care and insurance pressures have exerted an influence on health care in general and on mental health care in particular, resulting in briefer treatments. Concerns about the costs of health care have led to the growth of managed care organizations. The aim of these organizations has been to decrease costs and limit treatment durations. Despite the many problems associated with managed care, including bureaucratic delays, interference in the therapeutic relationship, and a focus on profits, this model of care delivery has produced greater accountability and more concrete treatment planning.

Although brief psychotherapy has much in common with long-term psychotherapy, there are major differences. Aside from the obvious difference in length of treatment, the practice of brief psychotherapy has special requirements. An essential element of brief treatment is the stance of the therapist, which must be active. The pressure of time requires the therapist to intervene rapidly to promote an unfolding of the patient's problems and history in order to develop a clear case formulation. Goals need to be clearly specified and may be more circumscribed than in lengthier treatments. In all psychotherapies, the therapeutic alliance plays a prominent role (Horvath and Symonds 1991); in brief psychotherapy, however, it is critical. If the therapeutic alliance becomes problematic or negative, it must be addressed and repaired relatively quickly, or therapy may fail. Although motivating the patient's interest in and commitment to psychotherapy is vital in all treatments, it is especially crucial to the rapid resolution of problems in brief psychotherapy.

Evolution of Brief Psychotherapy

Brief psychotherapy is as old as psychotherapy in general. Its history begins with the work of Sigmund Freud, who in his early writings emphasized the importance of a complete diagnosis, a thorough psychodynamic understanding of patient symptomatology, and the use of active interpretation.

In the early 1900s, Freud's treatment durations tended to be brief. In 1910 he treated the composer Gustav Mahler in an unusual therapeutic encounter: a single "session" that lasted 4 hours as they strolled the quays and canals of Leyden in Holland near which Freud vacationed (Jones 1955). Mahler had consulted Freud after a period of severe marital difficulties with his wife, Alma, that climaxed in a transient decompensation. The "session" appears to have been successful, as Mahler emerged from the meeting integrated, tranquil, and reassured with regard to his fears that Alma would abandon him. An indication of the treatment's positive effects was that Mahler was able to return to rehearsals for his massive Eighth Symphony (S. Feder, personal communication, July 1999). Freud also treated the conductor Bruno Walter in six sessions (Walter 1946).

At that time, the typical duration of psychoanalysis was only 6 to 9 months. Gradually, however, durations increased to many years. Part of the reason for this change may have been that Freud shifted away from the cathartic method to free association. In the cathartic method, Freud placed his hands on the patient's forehead and focused him or her on the issue being explored. The analyst's approach shifted from active to abstinent, and the patient was asked to free associate. The switch from a focused approach to free association led to a more roundabout and time-consuming treatment.

Another reason for Freud's turn to long-term treatment was his interest in gaining scientific knowledge. He believed that longer treatments would yield significantly more data about the mind. Paradoxically, an interesting development in the area of psychotherapy research has been the extensive use of brief treatment for research purposes, whereas relatively little research has been conducted with long-term treatment.

Several of Freud's contemporaries continued to be interested in briefer treatments. Sandor Ferenczi (1921/1980) advocated an active therapy in which the therapist at times would direct the patient either to avoid or to perform certain behaviors. Ferenczi's use of active techniques in the analysis of phobic patients to help them perform avoided tasks anticipated current behavioral treatments. Ferenczi also was interested in the interaction between therapist and patient and can be considered a pioneer in relational or interpersonal psychoanalytic approaches.

Otto Rank (1929/1973), emphasizing the birth trauma, attachment, and separation, advocated setting a time limit on analysis to enable the clinician to work on problems of separation. Rank also stressed the importance of "mobilizing the patient's will to change," a concept related to what we now call motivation.

Ferenczi and Rank, in their seminal work *The Development of Psychoanalysis* (1925), raised a number of important points that not only are timely today but also are central to several brief psychodynamic treatments as they are currently practiced. They argued that intellectual knowledge without affect serves as a resistance, and wrote: "[T]he actual effective remedy must be sought in properly connecting the affects with the intellectual sphere" (Ferenczi and Rank 1925/1956, p. 51). These authors also felt that the therapist should strive to keep some degree of emotional tension during each session. Change, they believed, comes about through a combination of affect and intellectual understanding of the original conflict in the transference.

In 1946, Franz Alexander and Thomas French's *Psychoanalytic Psychotherapy* was published. In this work, the authors examined classical psychoanalytic thought and challenged a number of traditional beliefs, including 1) the idea that the depth of treatment is related to the length of therapy and the session frequency; 2) the therapeutic value of regression; and 3) the notion that brief therapy produces negligible results in comparison with long-term treatment, which yields lasting and significant change. Alexander and French also questioned the value of emphasizing an intellectual rather than an affective focus. Their remarkable concept of the "corrective emotional experience" highlights the importance of emotional experience in treatment. According to this model, a corrective emotional experience takes place when the patient is exposed (with the therapist in the transference, and under more favorable circumstances than in the past) to emotional situations that he or she previously could not handle or found traumatic. These authors explained that "because the therapist's attitude is different from that of the authoritative person of the past, he [or she] gives the patient an opportunity to face again and again, under more favorable circumstances, those emotional situations which were formerly unbearable and to deal with them in a manner different from the old" (Alexander and French 1946, p. 67). Although some were critical of Alexander and French's model and accused them of playing roles in an artificial manner, we would assert that their basic concept is sound. Providing a corrective emotional experience without contrivance may be one of the major factors in producing a positive outcome.

In his 1933 book *Character Analysis*, Wilhelm Reich examined character formation and the development of various characterological patterns

(Reich 1933/1949). The book led to major changes in psychotherapeutic technique—in particular, a shift from free association to exploration of characterological or personality defenses used by patients to protect against unconscious material. Habib Davanloo (1980) adapted Reich's character analysis to create a technique that he called defense analysis. In this approach, the therapist consistently confronts defensive behavior until the character armor gives way to an affective breakthrough that is generally accompanied by the emergence of unconscious material.

World War II brought the need for crisis intervention and thus briefer therapies, particularly for soldiers exposed to battlefield conditions. The emphasis was on rapid intervention while facilitating release of affect for conditions such as combat neurosis or transient disorganization due to battle fatigue or injury, to enable soldiers to return to the battlefield.

Also notable in the 1940s was Eric Lindemann's (1944) work with survivors of the Coconut Grove fire in Boston, in which many people died. A number of the survivors of this tragic event suffered from acute grief and an inability to cope with their bereavement. These individuals and their family members were helped to do the necessary "grief work," begin the mourning process, and experience their loss. Lindemann also described normal and morbid grief, contrasting the two. His contribution is particularly important, because many patients seen in psychotherapy suffer from pathological or incomplete mourning and need to be given the opportunity to adapt to their loss as they complete the mourning process.

In the 1960s, interest in crisis intervention emerged in conjunction with the community mental health movement. This movement contributed to the development of short-term therapy approaches based on the belief that treatment should be available to large numbers of individuals with mental illness. The community mental health movement fostered the development of many innovative approaches, including a number of time-limited psychotherapies.

At about the same time, pioneers such as Mann, Sifneos, Malan, and Davanloo began to develop short-term dynamic psychotherapies designed for specific patient populations. James Mann's (1973, 1991) *time-limited psychotherapy* is particularly useful with individuals for whom separation and loss are central issues. In this 12-session treatment, exploration of and working through separation and loss are facilitated by the focus on termination.

Mann's theory of treatment was connected to the individual's conflict about time. On the one hand, there is a sense of "timelessness, infinite time, immortality, and the omnipotent fantasies of childhood." On the other, there is "time, finite time, reality, and death" (Mann 1973, p. 10). Applying Mann's formulation, we can summarize his ideas as follows:

1. Time is intimately connected to mortality.
2. The individual's earliest sense of time is connected to the idea that the child is omnipotent and fused with his or her mother with a sense of timelessness and immortality, or "child time."
3. The developmental task of the individual is to recognize and come to accept that time is finite and that reality and death must be accepted. Mann called the recognition and acceptance of reality and death "adult time."

Mann's time-limited psychotherapy is a psychoanalytic treatment in which the therapist defines the central issue and provides a setting that enables the patient to experience the normal maturational stages of development associated with time. In a sense, Mann's time-limited psychotherapy, with its focus on loss, is derived from Rank's work.

In the late 1960s, Peter Sifneos (1972, 1979) developed a form of psychodynamic psychotherapy that he called *short-term anxiety-provoking psychotherapy (STAPP)*. This treatment is targeted at patients suffering from anxiety, phobias, obsessive symptomatology, depression, and a variety of interpersonal problems. Sifneos originated the idea of using selection criteria as the basis for accepting patients into treatment. Among his criteria were a circumscribed chief complaint, at least one meaningful relationship in childhood, an ability to interact flexibly with the therapist, psychological mindedness, and motivation for change. Sifneos' use of selection criteria can be considered a beginning in the pursuit of differential therapeutics for psychiatric disorders. Ideally, the type of psychotherapy used should be tailored to the individual being treated, based on an understanding not only of diagnosis and symptomatology but also of personality and character structure. Unfortunately, Sifneos' selection criteria exclude a majority of patients, making it difficult to find suitable individuals for this treatment.

Sifneos' approach includes selection of a focus and use of anxiety-provoking confrontation and active interpretation. Behavioral indicators of resistance are addressed. Confrontation and clarification are used to help the patient experience his or her transference feelings. A positive therapeutic relationship is maintained throughout the treatment. The therapist does not address character traits such as masochism, excessive passivity, and dependence, because doing so can give rise to therapeutic complications and thus extend the length of treatment.

David Malan (1963, 1976, 1979), working at the same time as Sifneos, conducted a number of detailed studies at the Tavistock Clinic in England on the outcome of psychoanalytically based brief psychotherapy. He reported that important and lasting changes, both symptomatic and psychodynamic, could be accomplished in patients with severe characterological psychopathology. Malan's findings revealed that interpretations linking the therapist with significant figures in the patient's past correlated with positive treatment outcomes. He also reported that initial motivation and maintenance of an agreed-upon focus correlated with success in brief psychotherapy. Unfortunately, Malan's research had a number of methodological problems, including the lack of a control group and the use of therapist notes rather than audiovisual recordings. William Piper and colleagues (1986, 1991) were able to support many of Malan's findings, including the efficacy of Malan's psychotherapy and the importance of a focal approach and of patient motivation. However, they could not replicate the finding that interpretations linking the therapist with significant figures in the patient's past correlated with positive therapeutic outcomes.

Patients were selected for Malan's studies on the basis of clinical factors similar to Sifneos' criteria with the addition of the response of the patient to the therapist's active early interpretation of impulse and feeling, which Malan called "trial interpretation." Malan also developed exclusionary criteria for patient selection; among these were previous serious suicide attempts and drug use.

Malan employed the standard techniques of analytically oriented expressive psychotherapy, such as clarification and confrontation of defense, interpretation of wishes and impulses, and emphasis on transference interpretations and their linkage with parental figures. In addition, Malan stressed the use of a focused approach throughout treatment.

Davanloo (1980), working in Montreal, developed a short-term dynamic psychotherapy for patients with long-standing personality disorders. The selection criteria for this approach were similar to those used by Sifneos and Malan. However, Davanloo took Malan's idea of "trial interpretation" a step further in his technique of trial therapy. Designed to be conducted as part of the evaluation process, trial therapy would be used to assess a patient's response to confrontation and interpretation. If the patient responded with increased affect, particularly directed at the therapist, followed by production of memories or fantasies, his or her suitability for short-term dynamic psychotherapy would be established.

Davanloo's technical approach involves a high degree of therapist activity, meaning that the therapist relinquishes the traditional passive stance and becomes active and confronting when necessary. Emphasis is on use of the transference and maintenance of a therapeutic focus, which generally is an affective one. The transference is clarified and interpreted from the beginning. Davanloo used the *triangle of conflict* (Freud 1926/1959; Malan 1979) and *triangle of the person* (Malan 1979; Menninger 1958). Essentially, in the triangle of conflict, there is a focus on impulses and feelings, which are warded off by defense and anxiety. The triangle of the person also focuses on three points, all related to people: 1) individuals in the patient's current life, 2) individuals in the patient's past life, and 3) the therapist or transference figure. The treatment approach is interpersonal and requires the therapist to focus on conflict situations involving important people in the patient's life. The concept and use of these triangles will be more fully described in subsequent chapters.

The 1980s heralded the development of a number of new brief psychotherapies. These treatments were built on the work of the above-mentioned pioneers in the field as well as that of other prominent figures such as H.S. Sullivan (1953), Menninger (1958), Balint et al. (1972), Kohut (1971, 1977), and Gill (1982).

Lester Luborsky continued the work begun with The Menninger Foundation Psychotherapy Research Project (Wallerstein 1989) and formalized this work with a clearly delineated therapy (manualized) that he called *supportive-expressive treatment* (Luborsky 1984). Luborsky's treatment is based on the principles of psychoanalytic psychotherapy. Central to Luborsky's approach is the core conflictual relationship theme (CCRT) method, consisting of 1) the patient's wish, or what the patient wants from others, 2) how others react to the patient's wish, or how the patient perceives others, and 3) how the patient responds to the reactions of others. The CCRT is formulated within an interpersonal framework and focuses on relationship themes, which constitute the surface manifestations of the underlying core conflict.

Hans Strupp and Jeffrey Binder (1984) developed *time-limited dynamic psychotherapy*, an approach that relies on the use of interpersonal narratives to describe recurring cyclical maladaptive patterns (CMPs) that cause the individual lifelong difficulties. The CMP is a central pattern "of interpersonal roles in which patients unconsciously cast themselves; the complementary roles in which they cast others; and the maladaptive interaction sequences, self-defeating expectations, negative self-appraisals and unpleasant affects that result" (Strupp and Binder 1984, p. 140).

Jerome Pollack and colleagues (1991) developed a form of brief psychotherapy that they called *brief adaptive psychotherapy*. In this approach, the central problem is formulated by identifying the patient's major maladaptive pattern. Treatment focuses on the pattern as it is elaborated in the current and past life of the patient and in the therapeutic relationship.

Joseph Weiss, Harold Sampson, and colleagues (1986) devised a way of understanding patient communications that enables the therapist to map out core pathogenic beliefs within a time-limited treatment. These authors held that the patient is "governed by certain unconscious beliefs" (p. 6) and tests these beliefs in the therapeutic situation in order to disprove them. The beliefs are not impulses or defenses, but rather are derived from traumatic experiences. The patient repeatedly tests the therapist. This repetition is understood to be in the service of mastery of the original traumatic situation and/or series of real experiences in which the person's ego was helpless or weak. The pathogenic beliefs are disconfirmed because the therapist is neutral and interprets correctly. As a result, the patient feels safe. Formerly repressed memories become available to consciousness, and pathological beliefs yield to current reality.

The emergence of cognitive-behavioral therapies in the 1960s and 1970s, pioneered by Albert Ellis and Aaron Beck and elaborated by Barlow (1988), Mahoney (1974), Meichenbaum (1977, Meichenbaum and Goodman 1971), Goldfried (Goldfried and Davison 1994), and others, paralleled the development of brief dynamic therapy. Ellis, coming from a psychoanalytic background, began to question many of the practices of psychoanalysis and in 1962 developed a new psychotherapy that he called *rational emotive therapy* (RET; Ellis 1962). RET is based on an ABC model, in which activating experiences (A) interact with a person's belief system (B), leading to neurotic symptoms or consequences (C). Ellis described his therapy as consisting of "active-directive cognitive debating with emotive and behavioral homework…with a strong emphasis on…attitudinal change" (Ellis 1989, p. 8).

At about the same time, Beck (1963, 1967) independently developed cognitive therapy as a result of his work with depressed patients. He challenged the traditional view of mood alteration as central in depressive illness and instead focused on the repetitive, negative, and self-defeating thinking typical of depressed patients. Beck described a "depressive triad" of negative critical thoughts about the future, the world, and the self. These negative cognitions generally lead to dysphoria, passivity, and resignation. Beck developed cognitive therapy to target depressed patients' dysfunctional thinking and behavior.

Because cognitive-behavioral therapies are problem focused, they generally set a time limit in their approach to treatment. Cognitive-behavioral techniques are essential to an integrated psychotherapy approach and will be discussed in detail in subsequent chapters.

Interpersonal psychotherapy (IPT) was developed by Gerald Klerman and Myrna Weissman in the 1970s and 1980s for the treatment of depression (Klerman et al. 1984). IPT is derived from the interpersonal school of psychotherapy as delineated by Adolf Meyer and Harry Stack Sullivan. In its initial application, for the treatment of depression, IPT focused on symptom relief and improvement in social and interpersonal relationships. IPT addresses current problems at conscious and preconscious levels to promote mastery of social roles and adaptation within interpersonal relationships. In recent years, IPT has been modified to treat other mood disorders such as dysthymia, bipolar disorder, late-life depression, and depression in human immunodeficiency virus (HIV)–positive patients. In addition, it is being used for substance abuse, eating disorders, and a number of anxiety disorders (Weissman et al. 2000). Because an interpersonal focus is an important component of our integrated psychotherapy, IPT will be emphasized throughout this book.

Supportive psychotherapy is an integral part of most long-term and time-limited treatments. It is generally not thought of as a separate method of treatment, but rather as one end of the continuum of dynamic psychotherapy, which ranges from expressive to supportive techniques. Early papers on psychotherapy (Freud 1919/1964; Glover 1931) as well as more recent ones (Binstock 1979; Stewart 1985) denigrated supportive approaches. Alexander (1953) was one of the first to attempt to redress this negative image, and he did so by pointing out that supportive therapy requires as much theoretical background and technical skill as expressive psychotherapy. Paul Dewald (1971) described supportive and insight-oriented (expressive) therapies as two ends of a spectrum, both derived from dynamic principles.

Supportive psychotherapy has traditionally been a treatment for individuals with more serious problems. The past two decades, however, have seen an increasing interest in supportive psychotherapy, and a number of authors (Novalis et al. 1993; Pinsker 1998; Pinsker et al. 1991; Werman 1984; A. Winston et al. 1986; Rockland 1989) have described supportive psychotherapy approaches. Supportive psychotherapy has no exclusionary criteria and thus is suitable for a broad range of patients (A. Winston et al. 2001). Supportive therapy uses "direct measures to ameliorate symptoms and to maintain, restore, or improve self-esteem, adaptive skills, and ego functions" (Pinsker et al. 1991, p. 221).

Conclusions

The history of brief psychotherapy is long, rich, and diverse. The collective contributions of many of the authors discussed here serve as a foundation for our approach. In the next chapter, we address the developmental, conflict, and cognitive theories of human behavior that form the basis for our integrative approach to brief psychotherapy.

2

Theoretical Concepts

An Integrated Approach

Human beings are endowed with complex psychological structures and, as a group, function along a sickness–health continuum according to their level of psychopathology, adaptive capacity, self-concept, and ability to relate to others (Figure 2–1).

An integrated approach is one that is tailored to meet the psychological needs of each patient on the basis of his or her position on the continuum. The continuum is conceptualized as extending from the most impaired patients to the most intact and well-put-together individuals. Impairments consist of symptoms and behaviors that interfere with an individual's ability to function in everyday life, form relationships, think clearly and realistically, and behave in a relatively adaptive and mature fashion. Those individuals at the far right side of the continuum tend to function well, have good relationships, lead productive lives, and are able to enjoy a wide range of activities relatively free of conflict. At the center are patients whose adaptation and behavior is uneven, so that they have significant problems in maintaining consistent functioning and stable relationships. The determination of this point is accomplished by a thorough evaluation of the patient, which will be described in the next chapter. An individual's position on the contin-

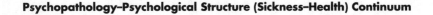

Psychopathology–Psychological Structure (Sickness–Health) Continuum

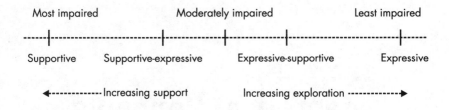

Psychotherapy Continuum

FIGURE 2–1.   Psychological structure/psychotherapy continuum.

uum can vary over time, depending on a number of factors. These include response to environmental stressors, physical illness, maturational growth, and psychotherapy and/or pharmacotherapy.

Placement of individuals on the continuum is associated with diagnosis. For example, patients with schizophrenia, bipolar disorder, psychotic depression, or borderline personality disorder generally lie on the left side of the psychopathology–psychological structure continuum. Patients with better adaptation generally lie on the right side of the continuum. These may include people with diagnoses such as Cluster C personality disorders (obsessional, dependent, avoidant), dysthymia, panic disorder, or adjustment disorders. In the middle of the continuum are individuals with conditions such as narcissistic personality disorder or mild to moderate major depression or hypochondriasis. Although the diagnosis can provide a general idea of where a person might reside on the continuum, the actual placement will depend on the individual's level of psychopathology and adaptation.

Matching psychotherapy technique to patient locus on the psychopathology–psychological structure continuum is of crucial importance. On the left side of the psychotherapy continuum are supportive approaches, which include cognitive-behavioral interventions directed toward building psychological structure, stability, a sense of self, and relationships. At the other end of the continuum are expressive therapies, which generally use an interpersonal/conflict model. Cognitive-behavioral approaches should be integrated with expressive therapy, since conflicts are generally complex and require many points of intervention. If problems in structure are significant, conflict issues are less important to work on; instead, the therapist needs to focus on repairing or building structure, relationships, and self-esteem. Patients with relatively intact structures generally will require work on relational and conflict issues. In practice, most individuals lie at neither end of the psychopathology–psychological structure continuum, but have both conflicts and structural problems. Therefore, the vast majority of patients will require work in both areas, generally beginning with relationship and psychological structure building, and then perhaps going on to address conflict issues.

It is important to note that comorbid conditions are present in many patients. For example, an individual may have more than one Axis I diagnosis, such as an anxiety disorder and a depressive disorder, and also an Axis II personality disorder. Different approaches may be indicated for the particular issues associated with each disorder. The anxiety and depressive symptoms may respond to cognitive-behavioral interventions, while the personality problems may require an interpersonal/dynamic approach.

That being said, the clinician's ability to use a theoretically integrated approach is essential in working with the complexities of people's problems. We turn now to a brief description of the theoretical foundations for an integrated approach based on the idea of a psychological structure/psychotherapy continuum. Although developmental, conflict, and cognitive-behavioral theory are described separately to maintain clarity, as previously indicated, these various models come together to inform the psychotherapy approach for a given patient.

Developmental Theory

Any understanding of individual development must center on the parent-child relationship and have the child's biological endowment as its foundation. The interplay between the innate capacities of the child, the biological and psychological capacities of the parents or caretakers, and other environmental factors will largely determine how development proceeds. The child faces developmental tasks involving issues such as 1) consolidation of early experiences, leading to establishment of basic trust as opposed to distrust (Erikson 1950); 2) emergence of a sense of the self as different from others, with appropriate boundaries (Mahler et al. 1975); 3) development of the capacity to differentiate affects (Jacobson 1964); and 4) establishment of satisfying and reality-based interpersonal relationships (Fairbairn 1952; Hartmann et al. 1946; Kohut 1971; Levenson 1983; Mitchell 1988; H. S. Sullivan 1953; Winnicott 1965). To the degree that early development is growth promoting, the child will develop a mental structure that enables him or her to negotiate future developmental tasks. Conversely, if the child is unable to successfully negotiate these tasks, he or she will tend to have limited ability to cope with what lies ahead.

Early infant dependency, coupled with the child's need for relatedness (Fairbairn 1952), sets the stage for the impact the mother/father or caretaking person will have on the developing infant. The mother is experienced as good or positive because she gratifies the infant's needs for relationship and care. However, at times she may not respond to the infant, thus frustrating its needs or wishes. The infant's developing inner world is shaped by repeated interactions, experiences, and traumas with primary caretakers and by its perception of these interactions. The infant develops a psychological object world that contains mental representations of both the gratifying and the frustrating mother and others. An object is defined as a mental image of a person. If the mother is too frustrating, damaging, or gratifying, the child may have a poorly integrated sense of self.

To further address the pivotal role of the caretaker as an interactive participant in the infant's development, we need to examine the concepts of *adaptation* and *fitting together* as put forth by Hartmann (1939/1958). Defining adaptation as the reciprocal relationship between the individual (organism) and the environment, Hartmann described the mutuality inherent in the mother-infant dyad. What the mother or caretaker brings to the infant's world is the sum of her psychic and physical being and all that she or he knows of the world. Ideally, the adaptation of mother and infant, each to the other, forms new levels of relational understanding and synthesis for both. Again and again the pair meet, each time bringing more to the relationship as a result of previous reciprocal encounters. Hartmann called this process "fitting together"—a synergistic interaction that adds more to the system because of the evolving relationship. This potentially enriching cycle is repeated continuously, enabling the child to learn about the world. The dialogue between the two—an interaction and mutual cueing (Spitz 1965)—sets the emotional "climate" for the pair.

Similarly, Stern et al. (1998), drawing on studies of infant development, proposed that the interaction between infant and caregiving environment results in "implicit relational knowing" (p. 903). Implicit relational knowing can be reorganized by "moments of meeting" (intersubjective moments), which can occur during a period of play or interaction, in which both mother and infant simultaneously understand that something new has happened between them (p. 908). This process continues throughout life in other relationships and has meaning for the patient-therapist relationship as well (see Chapter 4 for further discussion of the therapeutic relationship).

The child gradually learns self-regulation (Tolpin 1972) and comes to recognize certain urges as acceptable and others as threatening and problematic. An important aspect of self-regulation is the child's emotional life, which consists of experiencing, expressing, and containing a range of affects, including interest-excitement, joy, surprise, fear, distress-anguish, anger-rage, shame-humiliation, and contempt-disgust (Tomkins 1962, 1963). In addition, the child needs to develop increasingly adaptive and mature ways of coping with both inner and outer stimuli. The child's task is to adapt appropriately to his or her environment, which includes the immediate family or caretakers and society. Achievement of this task assumes a relatively benign family and societal situation, the so-called average expectable environment (Hartmann 1939/1958). The positive connection between caretaker and child, their attachment to each other, and the safety found in the relationship establish a secure base from which the child can go forth. The parent-child relationship plays a major role in shaping the child's development, laying the foundation for the individual's function in the world in a stable, cohesive, yet flexible way.

Among individuals who develop within the "average expectable environment" are those whose biological endowment creates significant inner turmoil, leading to maladaptive ways of perceiving, feeling, thinking, and behaving. An interaction between an individual's biological endowment and the environment will produce an episode of illness or maladaptive behavior or a chronic condition.

Achievement of mature object relations with a positive sense of self and other may be the individual's major developmental task. Relationships with others generally involve the interaction of early childhood experiences and the child's current needs/wishes and affects. A toddler needing reassurance from a mother nursing a newborn infant may feel rejected and abandoned. Another toddler, playing independently, may be content under the same circumstances. The temperaments of parent and child form the basis for ongoing interactions. The child's perception of these interactions, combined with needs/wishes and affects within the child at the moment of the experience and the child's basic temperament, form the template for character development. Predominantly positive interactions enable the child to develop a sense of the other that is enduring. An inner knowledge and mental image that another person exists in a positive way, even when absent or frustrating, is generally developed by the age of 3. This developmental milestone has been called *object constancy* (Mahler 1968). These early experiences tend to be repeated in current relationships and have important implications for the therapist-patient relationship. If a series of similar interpersonal experiences become associated with negative affects such as grief, shame, rage, or fear, a person may develop maladaptive ways of perceiving and interacting with others. In contrast, if these experiences are associated with interest-excitement or joy, an individual would more likely develop positive regard for self and others, which is predictive of better adaptation and functioning.

The emergence of the self occurs in concert with the development of object relations. Gradually, the infant begins to distinguish self from other. Kohut (1971, 1977) stressed the importance of the parents, whose special role it is to provide a delighted response to the child—the gleam in the parent's eye—that "mirrors back to the child a sense of self-worth and value, creating internal self respect" (Baker and Baker 1987, p. 3). A sense of self is promoted that is robust, cohesive, and positive and that provides a springboard for the development of ambition. The child also needs a merging experience with an idealized source of strength and calmness, from which goals, values, and morals may be formed. When both parents fail to provide these necessary functions, the child's sense of self is damaged and future development of a healthy sense of self is compromised.

Developmental failures spawn pathological conditions and determine their nature and extent. These conditions can be conceptualized as lying along a sickness–health continuum. For example, most patients with borderline personality disorder would be placed on the left side of the continuum, given that the disorder is characterized by a lack of self-cohesiveness and object constancy with severe fragmentation experiences. Individuals with narcissistic personality disorder would lie slightly more toward the center of the continuum if they have achieved object constancy but do not have adequate self-esteem. Patients with disorders such as schizophrenia or bipolar illness often will lie at the left side of the continuum (see Figure 2–1, at the beginning of this chapter). However, the latter two disorders have more of a biological or genetic basis, and the parent-child interaction needs to be understood from this perspective (given that illness in adulthood generally develops from a combination of environmental stress and an underlying vulnerability). On the other hand, even a child with an adequate biological endowment can be damaged by caretakers who are neglectful or abusive, and such a child is at considerably increased risk for mental illness as an adult (Brown and Anderson 1993). In addition, persistent emotional neglect or harsh, inconsistent discipline may produce anxiety and depressive disorders at a level of prevalence comparable to that observed in cases of abuse (Holmes and Robins 1987, 1988).

It should be understood that DSM diagnoses can only suggest an approximate placement on the continuum. A careful evaluation, including a complete ego-function assessment (see Chapter 3), will enable the clinician to establish a more accurate placement of each patient on the continuum. Although we think of ego structure as relatively enduring, conditions such as major depression, manic episodes, medical disorders, and posttraumatic stress disorder may temporarily influence a patient's equilibrium, displacing him or her toward the left side of the continuum. As such patients improve, they will gradually move back toward the right side of the continuum.

Individuals who have achieved a developmental level characterized by object constancy and a positive regard for self and others tend to have predominantly conflictual problems, which, in our paradigm, places them on the right side of the continuum. Although it is not unusual for such individuals to have developmental problems related to separation and loss, those problems will not be of the magnitude seen in patients with developmental deficits. In the next section we describe the major concepts associated with conflict theory, which generally is applied more to patients on the right side of the continuum.

Conflict Theory

Psychological conflict refers to a struggle or tension within an individual or between the individual and the outside world. Conflict may have its roots in unresolved infantile struggles that have been aroused by something occurring in the adult's current life. Within the individual, we conceptualize the struggle or conflict as occurring between various agencies of the mind or psychic apparatus. This discussion is derived from Freud's (1923/1961) structural model, which postulated the psychic apparatus as consisting of id, ego, and superego. Although, as originally described, the *id* related to the sexual and aggressive drives, more recent work (Emde 1992; Stern 1985; Tomkins 1992) connects it with the needs and wishes of the developing infant vis-à-vis the caretaker. The *ego* is conceptualized as having the executive functions of the personality. These functions include object relations (quality of relationships with significant others and self-concept), defenses, affects, impulse control, reality testing, and a number of autonomous functions such as thinking, perception, memory, and motility. The *superego* is viewed as containing two basic functions: the ego ideal and a system of values or morals. The *ego ideal* contains an individual's aspirations, hopes, and internalized view of self, and the *value system* includes conscience and ethical considerations.

The conflict model of the mind relies on the above structural theory. Fundamental to the conflict model's operation is the concept of a dynamic unconscious. Although predominantly unconscious, conflicts can also be observed through behavior, thoughts, and symptoms. Conflicts arise when wishes, thoughts, affects, or fantasies "come into conflict with internal or external prohibitions; the ego is threatened and produces signal anxiety; defenses are mobilized and the conflict is resolved via compromise formations in symptoms, character changes, or adaptation.... The manifestations of conflict vary according to developmental level, the nature of the psychopathology and cultural factors contributing to the makeup of the superego" (Moore and Fine 1990, p. 44). Individuals attempt to resolve both inner and outer conflicts and stresses in order to mediate the unpleasant affects associated with anxiety and depression and may use any means of achieving pleasure and avoiding painful affects. Psychopathology originates from the desire to ward off the painful affects of anxiety and depression that are derived from feelings of guilt or grief. According to Moore and Fine (1990), "[p]sychic conflict or intrapsychic conflict refers to struggle among incompatible forces or structures within the mind, external conflict is that between the individual and aspects of the outside world" (p. 44).

Thus, a conflict has three basic components: 1) a need/wish or affect, 2) anxiety, and 3) defense. An affect, impulse, or wish is a desire that expresses an underlying need or emotion. Examples are the wish to be cared for or loved, the need for admiration, the wish to be strong and powerful or independent, and the impulse to lash out or physically hurt someone. Anxiety is an affect characterized by an internal sensation of fear or dread, often coupled with thoughts that something unpleasant is about to happen. A sense of helplessness accompanies the feeling, and the danger is often nonspecific. Anxiety is frequently attended by an aroused physiological state consisting of heightened awareness, rapid heartbeat, sweating, muscle tightening, and restlessness.

> Alice, a 20-year-old woman, came to treatment several weeks before her wedding suffering from paralyzing anxiety. She described the anxiety as an inner sensation of fear along with an inability to take deep breaths, a tightening of the muscles in her chest, and a feeling of butterflies in her stomach.

When anxiety is barely perceptible, it may act as a signal of impending danger and prevent the painful feeling or emerging wishes from entering consciousness.

The concept of defense is central to dynamic psychotherapy. Defenses are psychological mechanisms mediating between a person's wishes, needs, thoughts, and feelings and both internal prohibitions and the external world. Although primarily unconscious, defenses can also be conscious, operating automatically. They generally consist of patterned responses, in the sense that individuals tend to use or experience the same kind of behavior, thoughts, or feelings in response to perceived danger. Defense mechanisms can come into play regardless of whether conflict is initiated internally or externally. They serve to ward off or push back the unpleasant affects of anxiety or depression associated with guilt or grief. Defenses may be adaptive, helping the individual to cope with internal and external difficulties or stressors. They can also be maladaptive, restricting, limiting, or inhibiting the individual's ability to function optimally and causing painful symptoms, which also limits functioning.

> William, a 36-year-old man, entered treatment complaining of severe anxiety and an inability to sustain a relationship with a woman. His anxiety would heighten as the relationship deepened. He ended each relationship by emotionally distancing (*defense*) and devaluing (*defense*) the woman he was involved with.

This example illustrates how patterned defenses (distancing and devaluing) are used repetitively to avoid anxiety engendered by close relationships.

A conflict not unusual in adolescents is illustrated in the following vignette:

> Steven, a 13-year-old boy, has a wish to be close to a girl in his class. He becomes anxious and withdraws from girls, spending more time in athletic endeavors with male friends. This is a partially adaptive solution occurring outside of the boy's awareness. The conflict involves the desire or impulse to be close to the girl in his class, anxiety is experienced, and the defenses of repression, withdrawal, and turning to another socially acceptable activity follow.

Most dynamically oriented time-limited psychotherapies use the concept of a *central* or *core conflict* (Davanloo 1980; Luborsky 1977; Malan 1963, 1979; Mann 1973; Pollack et al. 1991; Sifneos 1972; Strupp and Binder 1984). We believe that this is a necessary approach for all brief psychotherapies. If the therapist maintains a focus within the core conflict, a brief approach is facilitated. The core conflict concept provides an organizing framework for treatment, because both patient and therapist are in agreement about the conflict's centrality in the patient's life.

> William, the 36-year-old man described earlier, repeatedly ended relationships with women by using a variety of excuses. His core conflict involved the fear that his father would negatively judge the woman he chose and the wish to retain his mother as the primary woman in his life. Whenever Wil-

liam started to become close to a woman, he became anxious and ended the relationship. He developed the repetitive fantasy that he would find the perfect woman who would be acceptable to his father and mother, thus ensuring that he would never find an appropriate partner.

The central conflict is often revealed from repetitive fantasies. Arlow (1969, p. 44) stated that the "traumatic events of the past become part of fantasy thinking and as such exert a never ending dynamic effect." This suggests that fantasies from early life tend to endure with only insignificant changes. Arlow (1969, p. 47) used a literary analogy: "One could say the plot line of the fantasy remains the same although the characters and the situation may vary." This is another way of saying that people develop conflicts early in life that are expressed in fantasy as well as in behavior. The central conflict, fantasies, and behavior retain the same basic theme and are played out with significant people throughout an individual's life.

Cognitive Theory

In addition to developmental and conflict theories, cognitive theory is important for an integrated approach to treatment. Cognitive-behavioral techniques are an indispensable part of supportive therapy and can be used with patients in either supportive or expressive treatment for targeted problems such as panic, depression, phobias, obsessive-compulsive symptoms, and dysfunctional thinking.

Generally, cognitive-behavioral therapies share three basic premises (Dobson and Block 1988, p. 4):

1. Cognitive activity affects behavior.
2. Cognitive activity may be monitored and altered.
3. Desired behavior may be affected through cognitive change.

Cognition refers to the content of thought (what we think), the processes involved in thinking (how we think), and self-schemas (what structures our thinking). Ways of perceiving and processing material, the mechanisms and content of memory and recall, and problem-solving attitudes and strategies are all aspects of cognition (Neisser 1967). Cognition involves the process of interpreting and labeling an experience. The experience may be sad, threatening, surprising, joyful, fearful, irritating, or humiliating. Key concepts of cognitive-behavioral therapy include the schema construct, dysfunctional attitudes, automatic thoughts, and cognitive distortions or errors.

Cognitive structures or *schemas* are relatively enduring beliefs and attitudes that reflect experientially derived abstractions about one's view of oneself or one's identity (Kovacs and Beck 1978). These beliefs and attitudes are based on early learning experiences and are thought to account for problems in screening and encoding information. The concept of schemas can shed light on why people react differently to similar situations and why an individual may respond in the same way to different events. A schema enables a person to assess internal and external stimuli and then engage in a course of action. For instance, an individual may say "no" to opportunities to socialize based on a schema indicating that he or she is a loser and will not be liked. *Dysfunctional attitudes* are underlying assumptions that represent the content of schemas.

Automatic thoughts are thoughts or visual images that occur in an involuntary fashion, but are often at a preconscious level. Segal and Shaw (1996, p. 72) described three aspects of automatic thoughts:

1. Their instantaneous arousal in response to an external stimulus
2. Their unquestioned plausibility to the patient
3. Their detectability by attention-shifting, even though they are not always in the patient's focal awareness (hence the term *automatic*)

Cognitive distortions are systematic errors in the processing of information. Negative automatic thoughts and cognitive errors are reflections of self-schemas activated by events that are similar in content to the self-schemas.

DeRubeis and Beck (1988) described six types of cognitive distortions and automatic thoughts:

1. *Arbitrary inference:* Drawing a specific conclusion in the absence of substantiating evidence or even in the face of contradictory evidence. For example, a man who bought a new car began to think that he had depleted his family's resources, despite the fact that he had substantial savings and investments.
2. *Selective abstraction:* Conceptualizing an experience based on a detail taken out of context while ignoring more relevant information. For example, a woman in a middle management position who had always received outstanding evaluations from her supervisors was asked about a report she had recently written. She concluded that she must not be well thought of because her report was being questioned.
3. *Overgeneralization:* Drawing a general rule from one or a few isolated incidents and applying the concept broadly. An example of this is a student who performed poorly on a chemistry examination and concluded, "I'll

never do well in science and shouldn't consider going into this field or anything related to it."

4. *Magnification/minimization:* Assigning a distorted value to an event, perceiving it as far more significant or less significant than it actually is. For example, a woman who had her wallet stolen concluded that she was "irresponsible and not worthy of having anything of value."

5. *Personalization:* Attributing external events to oneself in the absence of any such connection. An example of this is a man who, when his boss passes him by without a greeting, concludes, "He doesn't like me."

6. *Absolute/dichotomous thinking:* Categorizing experiences in one of two extremes. For example, a mother whose infant grabbed and pulled her hair said, "My child hates me."

Cognitive-behavioral therapy focuses on how individuals make use of information to understand the meaning of events in their lives. Behavior and feelings are viewed as deriving from the nature and characteristics of thinking. Maladaptive behavior is believed to be the result of idiosyncratic dysfunctional thinking. Early phases of treatment focus on identifying negative automatic thoughts so that they can be changed. Later stages of treatment may address the underlying negative schemas.

Conclusions

A therapist using an integrated approach requires not only professional and interpersonal skills and knowledge but also the flexibility to apply these proficiencies differentially. How the therapist integrates and uses aspects of cognitive, conflict, and developmental theories should depend on the clinical assessment of the patient. In truth, most treatments contain aspects of many of the different theoretical elements outlined in this chapter. As a result, the therapeutic experience will be a unique one for each patient and for the patient-therapist dyad.

CHAPTER

3

Assessment
and
Case Formulation

Completion of an assessment and case formulation for a patient is an indispensable element of all psychotherapeutic approaches. The benefit to both patient and clinician cannot be overstated. One of the purposes of the evaluative process is to establish a therapeutic relationship and thereby enhance the patient's interest in and commitment to therapy. Another aim is to diagnose the patient's illness/problems so that an appropriate choice of treatment can be made. Although selecting the best treatment modality for a particular patient may present many puzzles, guidelines are available for making this choice. When a thorough evaluation is accomplished, the technical approach can be individualized in accordance with the needs and goals of the patient.

The organizing treatment approach for each patient should be based on the central issues emerging from the assessment and case formulation. For more intact patients (on the right side of the continuum), the organizing theme will be the core conflict. For more impaired patients (on the left side of the continuum), improving and enhancing adaptation, self-esteem, and overall functioning will serve as organizing goals.

23

Case formulation depends on an accurate and thorough assessment of the patient. Explanatory in nature, the case formulation is a statement about an individual's psychological functioning. An important but often unstated benefit of case formulation is the promotion of understanding and empathy for the patient, which in turn enables the clinician to guide and plan therapy effectively. It should be understood that the initial formulation is tentative and must be modified as more is learned about the patient during the course of treatment.

Accurate nosological diagnosis in no way illuminates an individual's ego-adaptive or -maladaptive elements, such as disappointments or achievements, the nature of the ability to achieve object relationships, and how the individual thinks about and interprets events. Nor does it explain the unique life history of an individual.

Psychotherapy in general, but especially time-limited treatment, must be designed to meet the needs of each patient by integrating different psychotherapeutic approaches. These approaches are derived from psychoanalytic, cognitive-behavioral, and interpersonal traditions. From the psychoanalytic tradition we first discuss structural, genetic, and dynamic approaches to understanding individuals. We then describe the cognitive-behavioral approach. Interpersonal and relational elements are incorporated into the four main approaches and within the case material. Although these approaches have always been described separately, there is a great deal of overlap among them, so there will be some repetition in the descriptions.

Structural Approach

A structural case formulation attempts to capture the relatively fixed characteristics of an individual's personality, which is understood within a functional context (in contrast with dynamic and genetic approaches, which are more content-based). Assessment of an individual's strengths and weaknesses and overall level of psychopathology helps determine the clinician's choice of technical approaches. A thorough structural assessment enables the clinician to determine, with some degree of accuracy, where to place the patient on the psychopathology–psychological structure continuum (see Chapter 2 for a discussion of the psychological structure/psychotherapy continuum).

Structural functions have been grouped together by using Freud's (1923/1961) structural approach of id, ego, and superego. These agencies refer to the inner life of the patient. The following description of psychological or ego functions is based on the work of Beres (1956) and Bellak (1958). It should be understood that these categories are not mutually exclusive and that there is a great deal of overlap.

Relation to Reality

Beres and Bellak described three components of an individual's relation to reality: reality testing, sense of reality, and adaptation to reality (Bellak 1958; Beres 1956). *Reality testing* describes an individual's ability to assess reality. It is impaired in the presence of faulty judgment and is grossly disturbed in the presence of hallucinations or delusions. *Sense of reality* relates to a person's ability to distinguish self from other, which indicates a stable and cohesive body image. Examples of disturbances in this function are depersonalization, derealization, and identity problems. *Adaptation to reality* describes how an individual handles everyday life, including relationships, work, school, and social situations.

Disturbances in relation to reality indicate significant structural problems that place the patient on the left side of the psychopathology–psychological structure continuum and should point the clinician in the direction of a more supportive approach. Relation to reality is a key indicator of structural deficits and should always be thoroughly explored.

Object Relations

Object relations refers to a person's capacity to relate in a meaningful way with significant individuals in his or her life. It includes the ability to form intimate relationships, tolerate separation and loss, and maintain independence and autonomy. It also involves the sense of self and the ability to form a cohesive and stable self-image without diminishing or overidealizing the self or other.

A patient's relationships with others form the foundation of the psychological functions constituting the structural approach. In brief psychotherapy, evaluation of object relations is central in determining a patient's placement on the psychopathology–psychological structure continuum. Patients who are withdrawn and not interested in others or who have narcissistic, highly dependent, or chaotic relationships generally will require a more supportive approach and therefore will be on the left side of the continuum. Individuals who have had at least one meaningful give-and-take relationship tend to be on the right side of the continuum.

Affects, Impulse Control, and Defenses

Affects are complex psychophysiological states composed of subjective feelings and physiological accompaniments such as crying, blushing, sweating, posture, facial expression, and tone of voice. The range of affects includes excitement, joy, surprise, fear, anger, rage, irritation, anguish, shame, humiliation, sadness, and depression. The ability to experience a wide range of affects at some depth needs to be evaluated. How well the individual differentiates between affects (as opposed to lumping them together into a single feeling such as primitive rage) needs to be assessed. Is there a wide variety and range of affects, and is the individual able to tolerate love, anger, joy, sadness, or humiliation? What are the predominant affects (R.S. Friedman and Lister 1987), and how regularly are they invoked?

The capacity to *control impulses* and to *modulate affect* in an adaptive manner indicates a well-functioning defensive structure. When impulse control is faulty, the individual may engage in socially unacceptable behavior, such as physically or verbally lashing out at others or making inappropriate demands. The ability to delay gratification and to tolerate frustration is another important aspect of impulse control.

Defenses mediate between a person's wishes, needs, and feelings and both internal prohibitions and the external world. Individuals tend to use the same kinds of behavior as patterned responses in reaction to perceived danger, difficult situations, or painful affects. Defenses are conceptualized as having both a developmental and a hierarchical organization. Three levels of defenses have been described: immature, intermediate, and mature. Some immature defenses are projection, hypochondriasis, acting out, sarcasm, and avoidance. Intermediate defenses include forgetting, intellectualization, displacement, and rationalization. Among the mature defenses are altruism, anticipation, suppression, sublimation, and humor (Vaillant 1977, 1986). Primitive defenses, poor impulse control, severe affective instability, and shallow affect are indicators of structural deficits that place an individual on the left side of the continuum and suggest the need for a more supportive approach.

Thought Processes

The ability to *think clearly, logically,* and *abstractly* should be assessed. The amount of primary process or primitive thinking is a good indicator of severe psychopathology. Significant limitations in the ability to think logically suggest the need for a more supportive approach as opposed to an exploratory one. Dysfunctional or negative automatic thoughts should be identified so that cognitive-behavioral approaches can be applied.

Autonomous Functions

Autonomous functions—perception, intention, intelligence, language, and motor development—are believed to develop in a relatively conflict-free manner (Hartmann 1939/1958). Although these functions generally are not impaired in patients on the right side of the psychopathology–psychological structure continuum, they can be affected in patients with significant psychopathology.

Synthetic Function

The *synthetic function* (Nunberg 1931) relates to an individual's ability to organize him- or herself and the world in a productive manner. It is the psychological ability to form a cohesive whole, or gestalt, by putting together the other functions and organizing them, so that the individual can function in a harmonious and integrated way.

Conscience, Morals, and Ideals

Conscience, morals, and *ideals* derive from internalization of aspects of parental figures and societal mores. Freud (1926/1959) conceptualized these elements as aspects of the superego. Severe impairments in these functions can interfere with the patient-therapist relationship. For instance, if a patient is not truthful with the therapist, achieving success in psychotherapy may be difficult.

The following vignette provides the basis for a structural formulation.

Structural Case Formulation

Bert, a 24-year-old man with panic disorder, developed the belief that his co-workers were saying derogatory things about him and wanted to hurt him physically. His relationships were characterized by an absence of concern for self or others, often putting him at risk. He used women to satisfy his sexual needs, abruptly leaving them with untruthful excuses. At times he became enraged with and was physically abusive toward them. His aggressive and violent behavior evoked fears of retaliation. He both used and sold drugs. The patient had a history of beginning schools and jobs and then quitting them when he encountered difficulties, blaming others for his failures.

This vignette illustrates a number of structural deficits. The patient has impaired reality testing, consisting of ideas about others talking and plotting against him. His adaptation to reality is poor, as demonstrated by his inability to work or to complete school. Relationships are conducted on a need-satisfying basis, without concern for others. Bert is often sadistic, but then becomes self-defeating and self-punishing. He exhibits impaired frustration tolerance and poorly controlled impulses, and his displays of rage may indicate a limited repertoire of affective responding. He uses immature defenses such as projection, acting out, and denial.

Genetic Approach

The genetic area of case formulation involves exploration of early development and life events that may help to explain an individual's current situation. Genetics are the genesis of the dynamics. Life presents many challenges, conflicts, and crises. These can be traumatic, depending on their severity, the developmental stage of the child, and the quality of his or her support system. Events or conditions such as loss of a significant person, separations, abuse, birth of a sibling, birth defects and developmental deficits, learning problems, illness, surgery, and substance abuse need to be considered as important in a child's development. A single event can have a traumatic impact on an individual, although often it is the day-to-day negative experiences that lead to significant conflict, psychopathology, and characterological problems. Examples of day-to-day events are constant criticism, devaluing, abusive behavior, parental conflict, and significant psychiatric problems. The genetic approach follows the development of the child from birth to late adolescence and/or early adulthood.

An example of a persistent difficulty or traumatic situation is that of a young boy growing up with a violent alcoholic father who is demeaning and at times physically abusive. Persistent trauma such as that caused by unresponsiveness of a parent may be more subtle and difficult to evaluate. For instance, a narcissistic mother may use her daughter for her own self-enhancement. She may ignore her child's real qualities, demanding behavior the child is either unable to deliver or can deliver only at considerable cost to herself.

Dynamic Approach

The dynamic approach concerns itself with mental and/or emotional tensions that may be conscious or unconscious. It focuses on conflicting wishes, needs, or feelings, and their meanings. In a conflict situation, an individual wards off or defends against wishes, needs, or feelings. The dynamic approach highlights the content of an individual's current conflicts and relates it to a primary lifelong or core conflict (S. Perry et al. 1987). In brief psychotherapy, the primary focus is on interpersonal as opposed to other types of conflict.

Dynamic formulation is concerned with meaning and content, in contrast to structural formulation, which is based on an individual's relatively fixed characteristics and functioning. The dynamic approach focuses on current conflicts, whereas the genetic approach highlights a person's developmental history and describes childhood and adolescent traumas and conflicts and their possible meanings. Childhood conflicts tend to be revived and relived in adult life.

A useful approach to understanding the dynamics of an individual, particularly the core conflict, involves the mapping of the central relationship patterns. An understanding of these patterns (Luborsky and Crits-Christoph 1990) requires exploration of three categories of interpersonal interactions: 1) what a person wants from others, 2) how others react to the person, and 3) how the person responds to others' reactions. These categories form the basis of the core conflictual relationship theme (CCRT) method, an approach that relies on "narratives, called relationship episodes, that patients typically tell and sometimes even enact during their psychotherapy session" (Luborsky and Crits-Christoph 1990, p. 15). The CCRT is composed of the patient's wishes or needs from others (W), how others respond (their actual responses as well as their responses from the patient's perspective) (R_O), and the response of the self, expressed or unexpressed (R_S). Understanding and using the CCRT provides the clinician with a central organizing focus. The CCRT method can be used differentially with patients according to their position on the continuum (see Chapter 4 for discussion of differential approaches to use of the CCRT).

The following vignette illustrates a dynamic conflict as well as its genetic or historical basis.

Dynamic Case Formulation

Tim is a passive 48-year-old man whose father has become increasingly debilitated and demanding, a state made worse by early signs of dementia. His father often telephones with complaints and demands, even though Tim has been consistently helpful. Following these calls, Tim finds himself wishing that his father appreciated him. He becomes anxiety ridden and often is angry with his wife and friends, later feeling guilty about his behavior. At work he has become increasingly anxious and perfectionistic and worries that his boss dislikes and will criticize him.

The dynamic explanation is that Tim has ambivalent feelings toward his father, consisting of anger and possibly a wish for his father to die, combined with positive feelings based on earlier experiences. He becomes anxious and defends against these feelings or wishes by displacing the anger he feels toward his father onto his wife and friends. The anxiety serves as a signal of unacceptable feelings. His boss is viewed as an authority figure and has become linked with his father, who is both loved and hated. In general, Tim is passive and avoids confrontation. He fears making a mistake and being humiliated. According to the CCRT method, Tim's wish (W) to be appreciated by his father can be identified. The response of the other (R_O) is lack of appreciation combined with hostility, and the response of the self (R_S) is displacement of anger onto Tim's wife and friends and feeling unappreciated. The genetic basis of Tim's current conflict is related to his experiencing of his father as being both highly critical and concerned and loving to him when he was a youngster. This early experience resulted in mixed feelings toward his father, consisting of love and rage with accompanying anxiety, guilt, and lack of assertiveness.

Cognitive-Behavioral Approach

The cognitive-behavioral approach addresses an individual's underlying psychological structure and the content of his or her thoughts. It is believed that the way in which an individual experiences environmental events and responds to them is greatly determined by cognitive processes. As discussed in Chapter 2, cognitive theory postulates that problems develop from the activation of underlying core beliefs by stressful life events. Prior experience determines how an individual will perceive an event, the meaning he or she will assign to it, whether the event will be attended to or remembered, and whether it will affect the individual's future functioning (note the similarity here to genetic/dynamic formulations).

Although case formulation has not been widely used in cognitive-behavioral therapy, models have been developed that are helpful in assessing an individual's problems in cognition (Persons 1989, 1993). Cognitive-behavioral therapy is initially directed at automatic thoughts, which are based on core beliefs or negative schema. Overt and underlying beliefs are closely linked and are expressed as thoughts, behaviors, and moods. Core beliefs are addressed later in the course of therapy. The cognitive-behavioral case formulation model has the following eight components (Tompkins 1996):

1. Problem list (including automatic thoughts)
2. Core beliefs
3. Conditional beliefs
4. Origins

5. Precipitants and activating situations
6. Working hypothesis
7. Predicted obstacles to treatment
8. Treatment plan

The above description of Tim will be used to illustrate the application of the cognitive-behavioral case formulation process. The *problem list* is a complete list of all of the patient's difficulties and presenting complaints. It includes the dysfunctional thinking responsible for the maladaptive behavior and disturbed mood. Tim's mood problems are anxiety, anger, and feelings of guilt. His problematic behavior is his inappropriate rage with his wife and friends. His automatic thoughts—"I am flawed" or "I will make mistakes and be humiliated"—lead to passivity and lack of assertiveness.

Core beliefs are hypotheses about the patient's self-schemas and views of others and the world. Tim's core belief is a pervasive sense that he cannot do anything right. This belief makes him especially vulnerable to the opinions of others and *conditional (if–then) beliefs*, which can increase his anxiety. An example of a conditional belief is the idea that if he makes a mistake, others will be very critical. The *origins* of core beliefs are early experiences, generally involving parents or parental figures. Tim's core beliefs appear to have been derived from his relationship with his overly critical father.

Core beliefs are generally *activated* by situations or events that are stressful or problematic for the patient. The deteriorating health of the patient's father *precipitated* Tim's current difficulty and brought him into treatment.

The *working hypothesis* forms the core of the cognitive-behavioral therapy formulation and incorporates the problem list, the core beliefs, and the activating events. Tim's anxiety, anger, guilt, passivity, and lack of assertiveness are based on his core beliefs that he can't do anything right and that if he makes a mistake, others will be very critical of him. These problems and core beliefs were activated or made worse by his father's dementia.

Obstacles to treatment need to be anticipated if possible. Obstacles in Tim's case might be reflected in the patient-therapist relationship. Fear of criticism can emerge in relation to the therapist and lead to increased patient passivity in the treatment situation. Tim may be reluctant to complete homework assignments because he fears that the therapist will be critical.

There are a number of similarities between the case formulation approaches in dynamic and cognitive-behavioral therapies. The concept of core beliefs and their origins is quite similar to the idea of the genetic formulation, which provides the origins of structural and dynamic factors. The notion of activating events in cognitive-behavioral therapy also is analogous to the precipitation of genetic and dynamic conflicts. Obstacles to treatment often are related to the therapeutic relationship, making this concept similar in both approaches. Cognitive-behavioral therapy adds a different dimension to case formulation and the treatment approach, particularly when thinking problems are present. Dynamic and genetic approaches do not involve a major focus on thinking, but the structural approach does evaluate an individual's thought processes.

A well-thought-out and comprehensive *treatment plan* should emerge from the case formulation. This plan should include goals and the types of interventions to be used (see Chapter 5 for a discussion of goals and interventions).

Initial Evaluation

The evaluation should be comprehensive and should be completed during the first hours of treatment, preferably in the initial session, enabling the therapist to understand the patient's major conflicts, psychic structure, and interpersonal functioning. The evaluation serves as a model for the course of treatment and provides the patient with a therapeutic experience from the beginning, thereby motivating him or her for treatment. The therapeutic experience during the evaluation promotes development of the therapeutic alliance, which many clinicians and researchers believe is a major factor in patient improvement (Horvath and Symonds 1991).

The evaluation should consist of an exploration of the individual's current areas of disturbance followed by a detailed past history. The presenting problems or areas of disturbance—including symptoms, relationship and self difficulties, work or school problems, substance use, psychological or physical abuse, and medical illness—are the first concern of the clinician and need to be thoroughly explored.

Generally, symptoms should be explored first, so that the clinician will be informed about the extent and depth of an individual's psychopathology. Significant psychopathology will draw the clinician's attention to the patient's structural deficits, which encompass psychological and biological factors. In the presence of severe psychopathology, such as hallucinations and delusions (which would place the patient on the left side of the continuum), the clinician should structure the interview in a supportive manner. Symptoms such as anxiety and depression should be explored before investigating relationships, work, or other problems. For example, if major depression is discovered early in the course of an initial evaluation, the clinician should not confront characterological defenses to explore underlying wishes and needs at that time. The degree of disturbance encountered at the beginning of the initial interview will determine how the clinician proceeds in that interview.

For patients on either side of the psychopathology–psychological structure continuum, a thorough evaluation of current problems and past history is essential. The difference will be in the technical approach—a more supportive one for patients on the left side of the continuum and a more expressive one for patients on the right side of the continuum. How to proceed technically will become clearer to the therapist as the interview unfolds. With some persons (e.g., a patient with serious structural problems, such as loss of reality testing), the appropriate approach will be evident from the beginning. With other individuals, structural deficits are less obvious, and more time may be needed to make this determination.

Once the current areas of disturbance are clearly delineated, the therapist should begin exploration of the patient's past history. One way to begin is simply to ask "Where were you born?" and proceed from there. Relationships with parents, caretakers, siblings, grandparents, and others of importance in the individual's life should be investigated. Issues such as separation and loss, geographic moves, trauma, medical and psychiatric illness, and family belief systems are central to understanding the individual. School history, sexual development and experiences, identity issues, and financial matters are likewise an integral part of a person's history. Previous psychiatric treatment, including the type of psychotherapy and/or any medication that the patient received, should be thoroughly explored. The patient's response to previous therapists always should be assessed, because these responses can alert the therapist to potential problems in the therapeutic relationship.

Trial Therapy

During the course of the evaluation, trial therapy is used (Davanloo 1980). Trial therapy involves the differential use of therapeutic techniques such as clarification, confrontation, interpretation, exploration and testing of automatic thoughts, self-esteem enhancement, and empathic statements during the initial session. As the therapist gathers more information, he or she adjusts the technical approach to the patient's structural level. The more intact the patient's structure, the greater the use of expressive techniques such as confrontation and interpretation, which are more challenging. The patient's response to these interventions provides an indication of the suitability of this type of treatment approach and further determines the patient's ego strengths and weaknesses. For patients who have structural deficits, emphasis is placed on clarification, self-esteem enhancement, strengthening of adaptive defenses, reframing, and other supportive interventions (A. Winston et al. 1986). Use of supportive techniques in an evaluation constitutes supportive trial therapy. Many patients with structural deficits will respond positively to these interventions. However, a number of patients with more severe structural deficits may respond poorly to both supportive and expressive techniques. Often, such individuals will initially do better with an "active empathic" listening approach (Winnicott 1965). In this type of supportive therapy, the therapist asks questions in an empathic manner and uses nonverbal forms of communication, such as nodding to convey understanding and providing simple verbal responses (including "Uh-huh").

Use of trial therapy enables the therapist to determine the appropriate type of treatment with greater accuracy and to provide patients with a therapeutic experience. As discussed previously, our integrated model combines supportive-expressive treatment with cognitive-behavioral and interpersonal approaches. If a decision is made to use primarily supportive psychotherapy, cognitive-behavioral techniques can be comfortably fit into this approach. In line with the supportive-expressive model, careful attention must be given to how the therapist conceptualizes and handles elements of the therapeutic relationship. If a decision is made to use primarily expressive psychotherapy, cognitive-behavioral techniques can be used both for specific disorders (e.g., panic, social phobia, depression) and in general to address dysfunctional thinking. To illustrate, we next present two case examples of trial therapy with our integrated model, one from each side of the psychological structure/psychotherapy continuum.

Case Example:
Right Side of the Continuum
(Conflict Model—Expressive Psychotherapy)

For individuals with good object relations and primarily conflictual problems (i.e., those on the right side of the continuum), the therapeutic approach is generally expressive. Our expressive model integrates ego psychological approaches with cognitive-behavioral techniques and includes an active exploration of the therapeutic relationship. In addition, as stated earlier, supportive interventions are used in expressive treatment, but the emphasis is on expressive techniques. The expressive approach is based on the work of such pioneers as Beck (1963, 1976), Davanloo (1980), Dewald (1971), Malan (1976), Mann (1973), Sifneos (1979), and Tarachow (1963) as well as recent work in supportive psychotherapy (Pinsker 1998; Rockland 1989; Werman 1984; A. Winston et al. 1986). In addition, Gill (1982), H.S. Sullivan (1953), Mitchell (1988), and Aron (1996) have made major contributions to our understanding of the therapeutic relationship.

In the expressive form of brief integrated therapy, the triangles of conflict and person are central. The triangle of conflict (Freud 1926/1959; Malan 1979) (see Figure 3–1) focuses on wishes/needs/feelings (W/N/F) that are warded off by defenses (D) and anxiety (A). In this model, when the therapist is pursuing a patient's feeling, he or she is at the W/N/F point of the triangle. Often, the patient will respond defensively to avoid the experience of a conflicted feeling. The defensive response is resistance when it occurs during psychotherapy (i.e., resistance toward the therapist and the therapy). Defense is the second point of the triangle. The patient also may respond with heightened anxiety out of fear of the conflicted feeling. Anxiety represents the third point on the triangle.

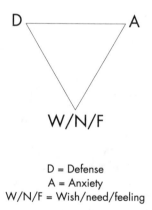

D = Defense
A = Anxiety
W/N/F = Wish/need/feeling

FIGURE 3–1. Triangle of conflict.

In the triangle of the person (Malan 1979; Menninger 1958) the three points all relate to people (see Figure 3–2): individuals in the patient's current life (C), individuals in the patient's past life (P), and the therapist or transference figure (T). Brief dynamic therapy, in its expressive form (i.e., right side of the continuum), is an interpersonally based treatment and focuses on conflict situations involving important people in the patient's life. The therapist's task is to work within the two triangles, using them to for-

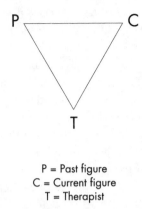

P = Past figure
C = Current figure
T = Therapist

FIGURE 3-2.   Triangle of the person.

mulate the patient's central conflicts. Defenses are consistently addressed, so that the patient's feelings can emerge and be integrated with his or her cognitions. The central conflicts should unfold as the therapist examines the patient's relationships in the past and present as well as in the here and now of the therapeutic relationship.

The following vignette, from an initial evaluation session, illustrates an expressive approach to trial therapy.

> The first session with Derrick, a 30-year-old single man, began with the patient's expression of hopelessness about his inability to move ahead in his career. He worked in the computer industry and described the kind of things he did. He then related a recent incident in which the program he used was not working properly. He was upset and disappointed because he could not complete the job. When the therapist asked if this was a fair example of what gets in the way of his success at work, he began a repetitive description about how difficult it is to get adequate help in the computer business. He complained that the support person at work, who was also a friend, ended up disappointing him.
>
> > Therapist: It may be that without realizing it, you get yourself into situations where you end up disappointed. Can you tell me who was involved with you in this situation, your support person?
>
> *The therapist highlights a maladaptive pattern and then moves it into the interpersonal sphere (i.e., the triangle of the person). The patient is asked to relate an example with a specific person. Ideally, the example should be concrete, not general. If there is a vague response, the therapist should address the defensive behavior, particularly when working in an expressive mode.*

Derrick: I called my friend, and he was late. Meanwhile, I tried to fix it myself, but I couldn't do it.

Therapist: You called a friend, who arrived late. His first name is?

The therapist asks for the friend's first name so that the patient's relationship with him becomes alive and personal during the interview, promoting intimacy between therapist and patient. Using first names of important people in the patient's life creates an atmosphere that can enable the patient to express the affect or emotion associated with that person and with the interaction being explored.

Derrick: Sam. I called him, and he said he would be right over. He did come, but more like an hour or two later.

Responds with additional information.

Therapist: And how did you feel toward Sam when he arrived?

Asks for feeling (F) toward Sam (C). The feeling (F) is a component of the triangle of conflict, and Sam (C) is an individual within the triangle of the person.

Derrick: I worked on it myself before he arrived, and I ended up causing more trouble. I was really pissed at myself.

Defensive avoidance (D) and shift to self-criticism.

Therapist: So you were angry with yourself, but how did you feel toward Sam?

Clarifies and refocuses on feelings (F) toward Sam (C).

Derrick: I was just upset that I messed up.

Avoids (D).

Therapist: Do you notice that when I ask you how you felt toward Sam about his lateness, you avoid answering my question?

Confronts avoidance (D).

Derrick: I was upset. Nothing was working right. After half an hour, I tried to call Sam again...I couldn't get him...that's when I messed up the computer. That's what I was thinking about when he arrived.

Avoids (D) and ruminates (D).

Therapist: Do you notice that you keep avoiding your feelings about Sam being late?

Confronts avoidance (D) again.

Derrick: *(He begins to stammer and responds in a hostile manner.)* Why do you keep asking me the same thing?

Therapist: You seem to be having some feelings about what's happening between us.

Addresses Derrick's feeling (F) in the therapeutic relationship (T).

Derrick: You're looking for a chink in my armor, my weaknesses.

Avoids expressing feeling (F) and attacks therapist (T).

Therapist: How does that make you feel toward me?

Derrick: It's annoying.

Expresses feeling (F).

Therapist: How do you experience your annoyance with me?

Asks for elaboration of inner experience of annoyance (F).

Derrick: I'm upset...I'm feeling tense, sort of jumpy.

Describes anxiety (A).

Therapist: Sounds like you're anxious now. Expressing annoyance with me causes you to become anxious.

Clarifies Derrick's expression of anxiety (A) and links it (interpretation) with Derrick's annoyance (F).

Derrick: I never like to show how I feel. When I get annoyed, I keep it to myself.

Therapist: You may be in the habit of hiding your feelings, but here with me it's important that we look at how you experience your feelings.

Indicates that habitual withholding (D) of feelings (F) will not be productive in the therapeutic work (T). Invites the patient to work collaboratively by using "we" (T).

Derrick: Yeah, well...I just feel annoyed. In my family we just didn't do that, especially with my mother.

Intellectualizes (D).

Therapist: Yes, we'll get to that, but let's stay with what you're feeling here with me. I can see it's not easy for you to be direct with me, and you've told me that in your family you've learned to keep your feelings to yourself, but let's see how you experience your annoyance with me.

Continues to focus on experience of annoyance (F) in the therapeutic relationship (T). Does not get sidetracked by information about mother (P).

Derrick: Okay, I feel angry, but I know you're asking me for a good reason...you're trying to help me. So I don't really feel angry.

Rationalizes (D).

Therapist: I realize that you know I'm trying to help you, but let's not avoid your angry feelings toward me.

Clarifies rationalization (D) and confronts avoidance (D).

Derrick: ...My neck and back are tight...I'm angry at you.

Expresses feeling more directly and the physiological concomitants of anger (F).

Therapist: Your ability to express your anger at me directly is important for our work together, even though it must seem different from what you're used to.

Supports ability to express feelings (F) directly and reinforces the collaborative nature of their work (T).

Derrick: It's different, all right...it's not what I'm used to.

Therapist: So now let's go back and see what happened. You thought Sam wasn't helpful, and you told me your mother was critical and that I was looking for a chink in your armor. Did you think I wasn't being helpful?

Clarifies and links Sam (C), Mother (P) and Therapist (T), a TCP interpretation.

Derrick: I thought, "This person is trying to help me, but at the same time I feel criticized." That's when I started to get angry.

Therapist: You felt criticized and wondered if you would get help from me, but it was difficult for you to express your feelings. Was it similar for you with Sam when you needed his help and he was late?

Links therapist with Sam and returns to explore Derrick's feelings (F) toward Sam (C).

In this evaluation, trial therapy of an expressive type was used. At the beginning of the interview, Derrick tells the therapist he is disappointed because he can't get "adequate help" at work. This theme may be a major one in Derrick's life, and the therapist should be alert to its appearance in the therapeutic relationship, which in fact does occur. The therapist recognized that Derrick was angry because he felt criticized, and helped him express these feelings directly. The automatic thought that others, including the therapist, are critical and not helpful is a potential obstacle to treatment. Early in the session, the patient became avoidant and ruminative when the therapist confronted him about his troubles at work. The triangles of conflict and person served as a model for the therapeutic work. The therapist redirected the interview into an interpersonal framework by asking to whom the patient turned for help. It soon became clear that Derrick had difficulty revealing his feelings toward Sam for being late. As Derrick's defensive behavior was addressed, he became angry at the therapist. He experienced the therapist as devaluing him and looking for his weaknesses. The therapist continued to work within the triangles of conflict and person by exploring Derrick's anxiety and defensive behavior, which he was using to ward off his anger at the therapist. Derrick revealed that he had learned not to express his feelings directly, explaining that doing so was unacceptable to his mother. However, the therapist maintained the focus on the therapeutic relationship, continuing to confront and clarify Derrick's defensive behavior until the patient was able to express his angry feeling in a clear and direct manner.

In this example of trial therapy, the patient was able to respond positively to an expressive approach that consistently addressed his defensive behavior. The therapist used a number of interventions, including confrontation, clarification, interpretation, and supportive statements. There was no evidence of regression or disorganization during the interview, an indication of Derrick's suitability for this type of treatment.

Later in the evaluation, Derrick's behavior with the therapist was linked to his relationship with his mother, who was an intrusive, needy, seductive, critical, and depressed woman. The patient's expectation that others, especially women, would be critical provides the therapist with important information with which to begin formulating the central conflicts.

Because all of Derrick's relationships with women were conflictual, he began therapy with a female therapist in a somewhat hostile manner. Establishing a positive therapeutic alliance under these circumstances is often problematic. The therapist recognized how difficult it was for Derrick to be with a woman therapist who was confronting his defensive avoidance. The therapist's behavior promotes a minicrisis designed to elicit an expression of meaningful affect. At the same time, the therapist's behavior affects the therapeutic relationship and must be addressed. It should be remembered that almost anything the therapist does or does not do affects the patient-therapist relationship. When Derrick became resistant during the session, his defensiveness was pointed out, and this enabled him to express annoyance at the therapist. Derrick's ability to be direct and truthful early in treatment without experiencing retaliation promoted the development of a positive therapeutic alliance. Attention to the therapeutic alliance from the first meeting onward is vital for successful psychotherapy. (For a more detailed discussion of the therapeutic alliance, see Chapter 4.)

As the evaluation proceeded, the therapist obtained a detailed history from the patient. Derrick's areas of disturbance are interpersonal problems, especially with women; dependency on his father; generalized anxiety; and work difficulties. He has problems forming intimate relationships with women. Although at first such relationships appear satisfactory, as soon as demands are made on him, Derrick becomes distant, hostile, and often sadistic. His last girlfriend dropped him because of his negative behavior, leading him to seek treatment.

Derrick has not been successful at work, where he continually procrastinates and often gets into arguments with co-workers. He tends to be passive with supervisors and others in authority. He believes that others should recognize his innate ability without his having to demonstrate his skill or knowledge.

Derrick grew up in a dysfunctional family with a chronically depressed mother and a father who was often away on business trips and preoccupied with himself. While often needy and seductive, his mother could become critical and devaluing. His father, although in general caring and supportive, could at times be harsh and cold. When Derrick was 13 years old, his parents divorced after many years of conflict. He believed that he was somehow responsible for their divorce. Derrick has a younger brother who suffers from depression, has great difficulty supporting himself, and tends to avoid involvement with Derrick. There were two previous psychotherapies; in both, Derrick abruptly left after a short period of time.

Case Formulation

Structural Approach

Derrick is an intelligent man with intact reality testing and sense of reality. He has problems adapting to reality in the areas of work and interpersonal relationships. His impulses are generally under good control except when he experiences frustration and becomes malicious and sadistic. Predominant affects are anger and anxiety, and major defenses are rumination, avoidance, and vagueness. Derrick's thinking is dysfunctional, characterized by the belief that others instantly should recognize his abilities and that women he helps should be devoted to him no matter how he behaves. Object relations are impaired, as evidenced by Derrick's inability to sustain an intimate relationship and his subsequent rage when women oppose him in any way. His sense of self is somewhat inflated, and his self-esteem suffers when he perceives even minor slights.

Genetic Approach

Derrick had been subjected to multiple rejections and slights from his mother, who suffered from episodes of severe depression. She was unable to care for him for long periods of time following the birth of his brother, 2 years his junior. She either was seductive with and dependent on him or was critical and spiteful. After his parents divorced, his mother moved to a distant suburb with Derrick and his brother. As a result, Derrick's relationships with his friends were disrupted, and he was unable to establish a satisfactory new social network. Derrick's father was a successful businessman who supported Derrick emotionally and financially but could also be cold and harsh. Derrick felt that he was in some way responsible for his parents' divorce that resulted in the loss of his father. Derrick's relationship with his father continues to be distant, although Derrick often asks him for financial help.

Dynamic Approach

Derrick's core conflict (based on the CCRT) is his wish (W) to be close to and loved and helped by others, especially a woman. At the same time, he also fears closeness with a woman. When others respond (R_O) with rejection or slights, he reacts (R_S) by distancing, avoiding, procrastinating, and behaving in a sadistic manner. His fears are based on his early relationship with his mother, who was seductive, dependent, critical, and hostile. His conflict about getting close to a woman also is related to his fear of being left with his mother, as he was when his parents divorced. His passivity with men is associated with his fear of being abandoned by a father who could be caring but also distant and harsh.

Cognitive-Behavioral Approach

The problem list includes Derrick's inability to follow through at work, his anxiety and hostility, and his inability to form an intimate relationship with a woman. His problematic behavior is his procrastination, his sadistic behavior with women, and the expectation that his father will continue to support him financially. His automatic thoughts are "When I get close to a woman, I will be criticized by her" and "I need to be passive and unassertive to protect myself." Derrick's core beliefs are "Others are critical of me and interested only in themselves" and "When I get close to another person, I will be hurt." These core beliefs are based on his mother's critical and seductive behavior, which resulted in Derrick's fear of intimacy, his procrastination, and his intolerance of criticism. Derrick's avoidance or fear of intimacy may also be related to his father's cold and distancing behavior. The loss of his current girlfriend was the precipitating event that brought Derrick into treatment. Obstacles to treatment include Derrick's fear of criticism and his pattern of precipitously leaving past therapists, which may interfere with the therapeutic relationship.

Diagnostic Evaluation

Axis I	Generalized anxiety disorder
Axis II	Personality disorder not otherwise specified (NOS) with obsessional, dependent, narcissistic, and sadomasochistic features
Axis III	None
Axis IV	Loss of relationship with a woman
Axis V	Global Assessment of Functioning (GAF) = 62

Treatment Plan

The evaluation and case formulation indicate that Derrick is on the right side of the psychopathology–psychological structure continuum, and therefore treatment should be primarily expressive. However, given that he has significant problems in object relations and work and thus is closer to the center of the continuum, supportive and cognitive techniques will also be needed. An organizing approach, based on Derrick's core conflict, is to focus on his wish for closeness with a woman; his fear of attack, criticism, or abandonment; and the defenses associated with this conflict. Expressive interventions will be directed at this core conflict and its derivatives, using the triangles of conflict and person. This approach should reduce defensiveness, integrate affect and cognition, and improve interpersonal relationships. The therapeutic relationship must be monitored so that a positive alliance is maintained, providing the patient with a noncritical, supportive relationship. Supportive elements will be integrated to address self-esteem, and cognitive approaches will be employed to diminish anxiety and correct cognitive distortions, which interfere with Derrick's relationships.

Case Example: Left Side of the Continuum (Structural/ Deficit Model—Supportive Psychotherapy)

For individuals with significantly impaired object relations and more severe psychopathology, the therapeutic approach is generally supportive, placing them on the left side of the psychological structure/psychotherapy continuum. Our supportive model integrates psychoanalytically based supportive approaches and cognitive-behavioral techniques. This approach is based on the work of Beck (1963, 1967), Ellis (1989), Foa et al. (1999), Goldfried and Davison (1983), Meichenbaum (1977), Pinsker (1998), Rockland (1989), Wallace (1983), Werman (1984), and A. Winston et al. (1986).

In the supportive form of brief integrated therapy, the major emphasis is on improving adaptation and ego functions as well as enhancing self-esteem. Because the objectives of supportive psychotherapy are different from those of expressive psychotherapy, the triangles of conflict and person (see Figures 3–1 and 3–2) are conceptualized differently. In the triangle of conflict, feelings are not pursued, anxiety is diminished, and defenses are strengthened. In the triangle of the person, the real relationship with the therapist rather than the transference relationship is emphasized and the therapist works primarily on present persons and current issues in the patient's life.

The following vignette, again from an initial evaluation session, illustrates a supportive approach to trial therapy.

Ella is a 32-year-old woman with interpersonal problems, anxiety, and difficulties with her work. Her history includes drug and alcohol use as well
as a brief hospitalization for suicidal behavior.

> Therapist: What is troubling you?

> Ella: I'm having trouble with everything in my life. I don't know
> where to begin.

*The patient is general, which could be defensive and/or a sign of disorganiza-
tion.*

> Therapist: Let's try to focus on one problem first. Where would
> you like to begin?

*The therapist attempts to explore one area by asking Ella to choose. Often, what
the patient chooses gives the therapist significant information. She may be direct and begin with the most important problem or be defensive and begin with
a less serious issue.*

> Ella: My boyfriend is hard for me to understand. I don't know
> whether to stay with him or not. He can't seem to get a
> job...just sits around a lot of the time. It gets me jumpy.

Presents a clear problem in current life (C) and her reaction to it.

> Therapist: You get jumpy; can you tell me what you mean by
> that?

Clarifies and explores.

> Ella: I get scared...my body reacts in all kinds of ways.

The therapist suspects that Ella may have an anxiety disorder. As discussed earlier, anxiety and depression, as well as other symptoms, should
be immediately addressed so that the therapist has a clear idea of the extent
of the patient's psychopathology. If significant psychopathology is present,
the therapist should employ more of a supportive approach. Severe symptoms may obscure or color interpersonal relationships, thereby complicating their exploration. If the therapist is aware of the extent of a patient's
psychopathology, exploration of interpersonal issues will be facilitated.

Therefore, at this point, the therapist asks a series of questions about
Ella's anxiety, including the following:

- How do you experience the anxiety?
- Is the anxiety with you all the time or is it episodic and how long
  does it last?

- If episodic how often are the attacks and when did they begin?
- Do you feel your heart pounding? Difficulty breathing? Nausea? Dizziness? Weakness?
- Do you feel as if you are going crazy or losing control over yourself, or that you might die from the attacks?
- Do you avoid situations because of the anxiety?
- Does anyone in your family have anxiety, panic, or depression?

The patient indicates that she has three or four attacks of anxiety a day, each lasting 5 or 10 minutes. Her heart pounds and she is short of breath, dizzy, and nauseated. She feels she is losing control and believes she is going to die. Ella has been having these symptoms for the past 3 years, but they have become worse during the past 4 months. Their worsening coincided with her boyfriend's pressuring her to get married. Family history reveals that Ella's mother has panic attacks with agoraphobia.

Having established that the patient has panic disorder, the therapist explains the diagnosis, indicating that a number of treatments are available that work quite well. The presence of panic disorder does not, in itself, determine the patient's placement on the continuum. A trial therapy will help establish the appropriate treatment approach.

The therapist then returns to an exploration of Ella's problematic relationship with her boyfriend.

> Therapist: A few moments ago, you were telling me about your problems with your boyfriend. Let's get back to that. What is his first name?

As mentioned earlier, it is important to obtain first names of important people in the patient's life.

> Ella: Yoshi; he's from Japan. As I mentioned before...he has an immigration problem and wants me to marry him. I don't know what to do. I want to help him, but I don't know how I feel about him.

Presents problem with a current figure (C).

> Therapist: Let's explore your relationship with Yoshi so we can understand what your feelings are. Tell me about him.

Obtaining a description of important people in the patient's life provides significant information and paints a portrait of the individual that helps makes the session come alive.

Ella: He's all right... he's tall and good-looking. He doesn't want to do anything much. He just sits around and mopes, watches TV, and worries he's going to be deported. He could do other things to stay in the country, but I keep worrying that if I don't marry him, he'll get deported, and it will be my fault.

Presents a portrait of Yoshi (C) and conflict about responsibility for him.

Therapist: If I'm understanding you correctly, you think you'll be responsible for his deportation if you don't agree to marry him.

Clarifies.

Ella: Yes.

Therapist: Isn't there some other way of looking at this? After all, you said there are other things he can do to prevent deportation.

Asks Ella to consider other possibilities.

Ella: Well, maybe, but I feel responsible, and also,... he keeps me company... and besides, without him I'm lonely. Sometimes he cooks and I like that, he cares about me, but then he gets pushy, telling me I have to marry him, and I pull back. Then I start to feel bad about myself... that I'm no good.

Presents conflict: wish (W) to be cared for, dislike of pressure with withdrawal (D), and then feels guilty.

Therapist: Can you give me an example of how that happens?

Explores by asking for a concrete example.

Ella: He keeps after me to marry him, saying he'll be deported.

Does not offer a concrete example.

Therapist: Is it difficult for you to tell me about a time when this occurred and you and Yoshi talked about it?

Empathically confronts Ella's vague response (D).

Ella: I can't remember a time.... I'm getting confused (*looks away from therapist*).

Defensive response (D), which may be regressive.

> Therapist: When I just asked you to describe a specific incident,
> you seemed to get confused.

Continues to confront defensive behavior (D) but leaves nonverbal behavior alone so that anxiety (A) is not increased.

> Ella: *(Silence)* . . . I . . . . What did you say? I don't understand *(looks away as if lost).*

Defensive behavior in the form of regression (D).

> Therapist: I was asking for an example of how Yoshi pressures
> you, but I see it's difficult for you to respond. Do you think
> I am pressuring you the way Yoshi does?

Clarifies defensive behavior (D) in an empathic manner and then attempts to link the therapeutic relationship (T) with Yoshi (C).

> Ella: I don't understand what you mean . . . that you're like Yoshi.
> No, you're not him.

Responds in a confused and regressed manner (D) with possible loss of object cohesion and differentiation. Ella's increasing confusion may be indicative of a misalliance.

> Therapist: You're right, I'm not Yoshi. I can see how hard it is for
> you to remember a specific incident with him. I don't want
> to add to your distress, so let's talk about the relationship,
> the positives and the problems.

Agrees with Ella in an empathic manner. Allows that too much pressure was used and shifts to a supportive approach in an effort to repair the misalliance, then asks for more information about the relationship.

The therapist began trial therapy by using expressive techniques, attempting to focus on a concrete example of Yoshi's pressuring Ella to marry him. Ella was unable to respond to the request and instead regressed, becoming confused. The interpretation linking the therapist with Yoshi was incomprehensible to Ella. Her response was concrete, and one may wonder whether she can work in the "as if" of the transference relationship at present. Ella's confusion may indicate that she has significant problems in differentiating objects and may not have achieved object constancy.

In this instance, expressive trial therapy produced a misalliance that the therapist attempted to repair by taking responsibility for causing Ella's distress. At that point the therapist shifted away from trial therapy of an expressive type to a more supportive approach, continuing to elicit information about Ella's relationship with her boyfriend. Ella described the things she liked about Yoshi, but emphasized that she did not want to marry him because there were many problems in their relationship. He was frequently ill, did not work regularly, and preferred to remain at home when Ella wanted to go out.

Ella: I like him, but he's not manly; he's more of a friend.

Suggests sexual difficulties with Yoshi (C).

Therapist: How are things between the two of you sexually?

Ella: *(Silence)*...He's not that interested in sex...

Therapist: What are your thoughts about that?

In a more supportive mode, the therapist generally should ask questions concerning a patient's thoughts rather than feelings.

Ella: I don't know. I don't know if I want a man sexually. I like it when he holds me, that's the best part of sex...I think I'm androgynous. I don't know...I get confused...sometimes I'm not sure if I'm a woman or a man.

Expresses gender confusion and a preference for being held.

Therapist: How do you mean?

Ella: Sometimes I feel like a man. My body doesn't seem to be my own, it's big and oafish, ungainly even *(in reality, Ella is slender and graceful)*. I feel good in pants, I never wear dresses. My mother only wears dresses; she never wears pants. I never wanted to be like her.

Expresses confusion, a feeling that her body is masculine, with the wish to be different from her mother.

Therapist: I'm interested in learning about your relationship with your mother, but for now let's stay with your feelings about your body. Do you sometimes think that parts of your body seem strange or different?

Continues to concentrate on Ella's feelings about her body rather than on mother.

Ella: Yes...sometimes my hands feel separate and large, like they're on their own; at other times I'm outside my body looking at myself (*appears anxious*). It's crazy...I think I'm losing my mind.

Expresses feelings of depersonalization.

Therapist: Having these feelings about your body can be very frightening. Do you also have similar feelings about the world around you? Does it appear strange, different, or unusual at times?

Empathic response followed by continued questioning.

Ella: (*Pause*) This is embarrassing. Sometimes the desk in the living room changes shape, the edges become pointy...or outside things seem to glow even when there's no sun...it's an eerie thing when it happens.

Portrays feelings of derealization.

Therapist: Does this happen when you become anxious?

Explores link to panic disorder.

Ella: Sometimes, but sometimes it happens by itself also.

Indicates that her depersonalization and derealization are not always connected with panic attacks. These symptoms may be incomplete or partial panic attacks or related to Ella's body image and identity problems.

Therapist: You indicated earlier that the pressure from Yoshi to marry him has made your panic attacks worse. Do you think that the feelings you're describing about your body and the world are related to Yoshi and the pressure you feel from him?

Interpretation linking pressure from Yoshi (C) with depersonalization and derealization.

Ella: That could be, I think I had these feelings before, but they are worse since he started pressuring me.

Responds positively to the interpretation. This positive response and openness with the therapist about her symptoms indicate a repair of earlier misalliance.

The initial exploration reveals significant psychopathology in the area of sense of reality and the self. Ella has identity confusion and ego boundary problems, as demonstrated by her sense that her body is not her own. The therapist elicited evidence of depersonalization when Ella described her experience of her body, and of derealization when she indicated that at times she perceives objects as changing shape and the world as looking different.

The session continued with an exploration of Ella's relationship with her mother.

> Therapist: You mentioned problems with your parents and not wanting to be like your mother. Can you tell me about your relationship with your mother?

Continues to explore relationship problems, using the triangle of the person, by asking about Ella's mother (P).

> Ella: I always wanted a mother like other mothers. Other mothers drive cars and can go places by themselves. My mother just stayed home, and she expected me to take care of her.

States that she longs for an active mother who is independent (W).

> Therapist: So you found it difficult because your mother was different. Tell me what your mother looks like and what kind of person she is.

Asks for description of mother, but loses an opportunity to explore wish for a different kind of mother (P) and the link to Yoshi (C).

> Ella: She's nice-looking and dark like me, but overweight and has trouble walking. She's pretty nice but is always asking for help. I think she's an alcoholic. She starts drinking around noon and can't get anything done.

> Therapist: And her drinking, how did that affect you?

Focuses on mother's (P) alcoholism and its effect on Ella.

> Ella: I'm embarrassed by her. She never cooked; there was hardly any food in the house. My father didn't care, he never was home, he worked late. We just took care of ourselves...they never made me feel good about myself.

Indicates mother's (P) lack of support.

> Therapist: You were on your own and had to manage because your mother wasn't available enough. Do you think she cared about you?

Clarifies.

> Ella: I think she cared, but she just couldn't do things. She didn't give me help, and it's hard for me to be on my own. She hung onto me…. I had to take her places.

In this part of the evaluation, the therapist employed supportive trial therapy. Ella was more responsive to this approach than to the expressive mode initially employed, indicating that supportive psychotherapy was the appropriate treatment and she was currently on the left side of the continuum.

The therapist continued the evaluation, gathering additional information. Ella is the older of two daughters and grew up in an intact family. Her mother was a dependent woman with panic disorder, agoraphobia, and alcoholism, and her father, a cold and distant man, was also an alcoholic and had many medical problems. The patient has a history of excessive use of alcohol and marijuana and occasional use of cocaine. Prior to entering treatment, she was hospitalized after a suicide attempt following the loss of a boyfriend. Ella has a great deal of interpersonal difficulty with men, alternating between clinging, needy behavior and distancing and withdrawal. When she becomes angry or disappointed with others, she dismisses them, stating that they are "no good." At times, she would form sexual attachments to women, and similar interpersonal difficulties would ensue. In her words, "I can be with a man or a woman—it doesn't matter."

There were periods in her life, beginning in adolescence, when Ella would cut herself with a razor. This occurred when her mood was anxious or down and she was feeling neglected by her mother or by friends.

Case Formulation

Structural Approach

Ella is a woman of average intelligence with intact reality testing. Her sense of reality is impaired. She experiences depersonalization, derealization, and gender and sexual confusion. She has distortions of body image, and at times her world appears strange or different. Her gender identity is not firmly established, and she views men and women as interchangeable. Object relations are based on need satisfaction, and she has not achieved object constancy.

Ella impulsively cuts herself or uses drugs when she has difficulty tolerating her affects (anger, anxiety, or sadness). Defenses used are forgetting, regression, splitting, and vagueness. Her thinking is dysfunctional, as exemplified by her misappraisal of her role in Yoshi's immigration problem. Ella has a somewhat harsh superego, with poor self-esteem, and would blame herself if Yoshi were deported.

Genetic Approach

Ella was raised by a needy, alcoholic mother who suffered from panic disorder, agoraphobia, and alcoholism. She was used as a caretaker and was expected to take over many of her mother's functions, even at an early age. Ella was exposed to her mother's irrational anxieties and recalls being prevented from going out with her friends. Her mother's neediness interfered with Ella's ability to separate from her and become autonomous. Her father, also an alcoholic, suffered from a number of severe medical illnesses related to his alcoholism. He was cold and distant with Ella. The patient's daily exposure to her parents' preoccupation with drinking resulted in feelings of neglect and worthlessness.

Dynamic Approach

Ella's wish (W) or need is to be cared for. The response of others (R_O) is to disappoint her or to be neglectful or erratic in providing support. At times Ella reacts (R_S) by becoming forgetful and vague, and her sense of self becomes fragmented; at other times she assumes the role of caretaker. Her wish is derived from feeling neglected by her mother and ignored by her father. In her current life, Ella takes on a parental role with her boyfriend. Her neediness leads her to pursue both men and women. Her gender confusion and inability to declare a sexual preference afford her an omnipotentiality of object choices. When disappointed by others, she eliminates them from her life and moves on, searching for a replacement.

Cognitive-Behavioral Approach

Ella's problems include interpersonal difficulties with her boyfriend, including her belief that she is responsible for his well-being; identity issues; substance abuse; parasuicidal behavior; and panic attacks. Her automatic thoughts are "I am responsible for the well-being of others" and "I need someone to care for me." Ella's major conditional beliefs are "If I disappoint others, I am a failure and of little value" and "If I don't have someone to care for me, I will not be able to manage on my own." Her core beliefs come from early childhood, when Ella was responsible for carrying out tasks her mother was unable to perform. The activating situation is her boyfriend's insistence that she marry him so that he can avoid deportation. Obstacles to treatment might arise as a result of Ella's propensity for acting out and either cutting herself or using drugs.

Diagnostic Evaluation

Axis I	Panic disorder
Axis II	Borderline personality disorder
Axis III	None
Axis IV	Pressure from boyfriend
Axis V	GAF = 50

Treatment Plan

Ella has multiple difficulties, including serious structural deficits, panic disorder, dysfunctional thinking, and interpersonal conflicts. The evaluation interview identified body-image issues and identity confusion, which may need an extended period of treatment to be resolved. Ella did not raise these issues as concerns, but instead stated that she wanted help with her interpersonal problems and panic disorder. A supportive approach with cognitive-behavioral and expressive elements is indicated in view of Ella's structural deficits, which place her on the left side of the continuum. Cognitive-behavioral interventions will be directed at Ella's dysfunctional thinking and her panic disorder symptoms. Interpersonal conflicts will be addressed with supportive and expressive interventions. Serotonin reuptake inhibitor medication will be considered if her panic disorder does not respond to cognitive-behavioral treatment.

Patient Selection

Patient selection for brief psychotherapy has generally been made on the basis of criteria derived from specific approaches. Innovators such as Malan and Sifneos developed criteria based on their treatments. For example, Sifneos (1972, 1979) delineated the following selection criteria for his short-term anxiety-provoking psychotherapy: 1) above-average intelligence, 2) history of at least one meaningful give-and-take relationship with another person, 3) ability to interact with the evaluator, as assessed by expressing emotion appropriately during the interview and showing some degree of flexibility, 4) presence of a circumscribed chief complaint, and 5) motivation for change.

Malan (1963, 1976, 1979) described similar inclusion criteria for his brief dynamic psychotherapy. He also provided exclusion criteria, which include existence of severe suicidal impulses, history of long-term psychiatric hospitalization, and presence of addictive disorders.

In addition to these criteria, Malan developed the innovative idea of trial interpretation. By this, he meant using interpretations during an evaluation to assess the patient's responsiveness to interpretive work. Davanloo (1980) took Malan's trial interpretation a step further and developed trial therapy. During the course of an evaluation, the therapist engages in psychotherapy to test the patient's ability to respond in a meaningful way. In Davanloo's short-term dynamic psychotherapy, trial therapy would involve challenging the patient's defensive behavior to enable the patient to respond with appropriate affect.

Unfortunately, in these systems of selection, the patient must meet the criteria or be rejected for the psychotherapy. However, an approach based on the psychopathology–psychological structure continuum and integrating cognitive-behavioral and interpersonal/dynamic models can accommodate a wide variety of patients.

The criteria for selection of patients for an integrated therapy of this type are broad based and inclusive. Many patients can be treated appropriately with a short-term approach. This is especially true if the integrated approach includes a medication option (see Chapter 6). The key issue in patient selection is determining which type of brief psychotherapy is indicated for a given patient. As described earlier in this chapter, treatment decisions are based on a thorough patient evaluation that determines the patient's placement on the psychopathology–psychological structure continuum. The continuum allows for the use of differential therapeutics to select the appropriate technical approach for a patient. It does not try to fit the patient into a treatment.

However, individuals with certain diagnoses will generally not benefit from brief psychotherapy. These include patients with disorders that require long-term supportive care and rehabilitation, such as schizophrenia, bipolar illness, severe recurrent depression, and anorexia nervosa. Patients with personality disorders of the borderline, narcissistic, schizoid, schizotypal, and paranoid types also generally require long-term treatment. Nevertheless, some borderline and narcissistic patients may do quite well with a short-term approach with a limited focus and can be offered a trial of brief psychotherapy. Indeed, after a successful brief therapy, many patients return for additional courses of treatment. This may be a useful approach for individuals with significant personality problems.

Conclusions

Assessment of the patient's problems, symptoms, and character structure is critical to arriving at a complete diagnosis, case formulation, and treatment plan. Trial therapy is an invaluable aid in the assessment process in placing the patient on the continuum. The case formulation should be broad based, encompassing structural, genetic, dynamic, and cognitive-behavioral approaches. We have illustrated this process by presenting material from an initial assessment of two patients from two sides of the continuum.

CHAPTER

4

The Therapeutic Relationship

People have undoubtedly appreciated the centrality of personal relationships from the beginning of time, but it took the understanding of the therapeutic relationship in psychotherapy to harness its potential for treatment. More than a century ago, Freud (Breuer and Freud 1893–1895/1955) became aware of the concept of transference, but it was not until after his treatment of Dora, in which she precipitously left therapy, that he recognized its importance (Freud 1905a/1953). He identified different types of transference: a negative transference that served resistance, and a positive transference of unconscious erotic impulses. Freud also described a second type of positive transference consisting of conscious "friendly or affectionate feelings" that were "unobjectionable." These friendly, affectionate, and unobjectionable feelings the patient felt toward the analyst were called "the vehicle of success in psychoanalysis" (Freud 1912/1958). These many years later, clinicians and researchers have found that the patient-therapist relationship may be the most important variable in successful outcome of treatment.

Two aspects of the therapeutic relationship are transference and the real relationship (Greenson 1967, 1971). The "unobjectionable positive transference" is a component of the real relationship and forms an essential part of

57

the foundation upon which all psychotherapy stands. Zetzel (1956, 1966) first used the term *therapeutic alliance* for the "unobjectionable positive transference," which was seen as an essential element in the success of psychotherapy. Greenson (1967, 1971) conceptualized the therapeutic alliance as the patient and therapist working together on a mutual task.

In this chapter, we divide the therapeutic relationship into three components: the transference/countertransference, the real relationship, and the therapeutic alliance. Although we believe that the three are intimately related and form a cohesive whole, we will discuss them separately for the sake of clarity. Transference and real relationship issues play a role in every transaction within the therapeutic relationship. At certain times transference aspects may be more important, while at other times real relationship issues may predominate. From this point of view, a continuum exists between transference issues and real issues that corresponds to the supportive–expressive psychotherapy continuum. Expressive therapy places more emphasis on the transference, while supportive and cognitive-behavioral treatments focus more on the real relationship.

The transference and the therapeutic alliance also are interrelated. Changes of transference/countertransference configurations over the course of psychotherapy will have a major influence on the therapeutic alliance. An individual's past relationships directly affect the therapeutic alliance in much the same way as they do the transference.

Some writers have argued that the distinction between the transference and the real relationship is a false one. For example, B. S. Kohlenberg et al. (1998) stated that "behavior is always controlled by both remote and immediate contingencies." Although this is also our view, we believe that the distinction between the transference and the real relationship remains a valuable one. Clarity and richness are furthered by maintaining this conceptual framework. Accordingly, in what follows, we will examine each of the areas separately and then integrate them.

Transference

Classically, transference has been described as a special type of object relationship consisting of behaviors, thoughts, feelings, wishes, and attitudes directed at the therapist that are related to important people in the patient's past (Greenson 1967). Most commonly displaced onto the therapist are attitudes toward significant people such as parents, siblings, grandparents, or teachers. Essentially, the past is revived in the present.

Transference reactions can be positive or negative. On the expressive side of the psychotherapy continuum, both positive and negative transference reactions are explored. On the supportive side of the continuum, positive transference reactions generally are not explored, but rather are simply accepted. Negative reactions must always be investigated, however, because they may compromise the treatment. In the middle range of the psychotherapy continuum, a flexible approach should be taken. The approach used depends on the patient's receptivity and ability to work in the transference.

The following vignette illustrates some of the strategies employed to address positive transference reactions at different points along the psychotherapy continuum.

Jay, a 44-year-old man, tells his therapist how much his relationship with his wife has improved since he has started therapy. He attributes this change to the therapist's interest in him.

In expressive psychotherapy, the experience and meaning of the therapist's interest should be explored. The therapist could say, "Let's examine how you experience and feel about my interest in you."

In supportive and cognitive-behavioral psychotherapy, the therapist, instead of exploring, would accept the compliment, conceptualizing Jay's statement as a reflection of the real relationship, and might say: "I'm glad to be of help to you." This opportunity also might be used to bolster the patient's self-esteem by adding, "Since our work has been a joint effort, you have to take some credit too."

The technique for patients in the middle range of the continuum is similar to the supportive approach, especially at the beginning of treatment. After the initial treatment phase, however, an examination might be undertaken of the meaning of the patient's statement, rather than the patient's experience or feelings about the therapist's interest. "How do you think my interest has made a difference in your behavior with your wife?" is a question that might be asked by the therapist. The patient's statement might also be a reflection of his need to please the therapist, and this issue may need exploration.

The choice between exploring feelings and exploring thoughts depends on the patient's placement on the continuum. Individuals with significant structural impairment experience difficulty examining feelings but are often able to explore their thoughts. Thus, a more cognitive than affective approach is indicated for these individuals. In the example above, the therapist understands that the patient's improved communication with his wife may be multiply determined. It may be that the patient's relationship with his wife improved because therapist and patient worked on communication skills; or that, unlike the patient's father, the therapist is not competitive, so there is less fear of retaliation within a safer environment. Another possibility may be that Jay's improved relationship with his wife is a defense against his yearning for and fear of closeness with a man. In brief expressive psychotherapy, transference-related conflicts of this sort are generally explored, in contrast to a more supportive therapy.

An example of a negative transference reaction follows.

Flora, a 63-year-old woman in brief expressive psychotherapy, tells her therapist that she has been confiding in her two sisters much more than she had in the past. The therapist asks whether she is having trouble confiding in him. Flora begins to speak hesitantly but trails off and becomes silent. The patient has defensively withdrawn. The therapist asks her how she experienced his comment. Flora acknowledges feeling criticized.

Although the therapist realizes that the patient's feeling criticized is partially fueled by early relational patterns in her life, the initial exploration begins in the here and now of the therapeutic relationship. In supportive, expressive, and cognitive-behavioral psychotherapy, negative transference reactions should be examined. However, in cognitive-behavioral and supportive psychotherapy, a more cognitive exploration would lead to the therapist's asking, "What thoughts do you have about my comment?"

The above examples illustrate transference exploration in the here and now of the patient-therapist relationship. It is preferable to fully explore transference reactions in the therapeutic relationship before turning to their origins in the past (Gill and Muslin 1976). In fact, Freud (1912/1958) indicated that although transference derives from application of a past relationship to a current one, the term refers to the present, to the current relationship between patient and therapist. The here and now of the transference relationship generally is compelling, immediate, and emotionally charged, enabling the patient to have a give-and-take experience with the therapist. Turning to the origins of the transference before exploring current manifestations of transference reactions may promote an intellectual process that is less therapeutic.

The example of Flora, the woman who felt criticized by the therapist, illustrates this approach. The therapist knew that the patient's negative transference was partly fueled by her critical experiences with her father; however, he remained within the here and now of the transference by exploring Flora's feelings toward *him*, the therapist. It is important to emphasize that if the transference is understood as an interplay between the therapist and patient taking place within an interactive process, the first line of exploration should be the here and now of the therapeutic relationship. The therapist, too, is a participant who is actively engaged with the patient;

he or she is not an entirely neutral person upon whom the patient displaces thoughts, feelings, and wishes. The therapist's history, character, foibles, and other attributes play a significant role in transference/countertransference reactions. In addition to being aware of how the patient experiences interactions with others and within the patient-therapist relationship, the therapist needs to monitor responses that come from his or her own personality (Aron 1996; Gill 1982; Levenson 1983; Mitchell 1988; Singer 1998). For instance, in the case of Flora, the therapist needs to understand why he asked the patient whether she was having trouble confiding in him. Did his question come from something personal and have little to do with the patient?

The nature of the interactive process occurring between patient and therapist is further described in the relational model of psychoanalysis (Aron 1996). Because the therapeutic relationship takes place in a social environment, the ongoing participation of therapist and patient creates new meaning and experience—a result of entry of the therapist into the patient's relational world and their mutual collaboration. A patient's maladaptive relational patterns will be repeated in treatment and will be worked out within the new object relationship created by and understood within the patient-therapist relationship (Bromberg 1991).

In expressive psychotherapy, it is appropriate to investigate linkages with past and present people in the patient's life (i.e., TCP [therapist–current life–past life] interpretations [discussed in Chapter 3]) only after a full exploration of the transference reaction with the therapist has been undertaken. Such exploration helps make the patient aware of the origins of conflicts and can delineate the core conflict. Thus, the next step in the above example of Flora would be an exploration of the patient's relationship with her critical father.

> Flora recounted a memory from age 6 years, when she had proudly demonstrated her reading ability to her father. She mistakenly pronounced the word *ear* as if it was "air." He criticized her pronunciation and walked away, leaving her feeling stupid and humiliated.

Working in the transference can produce memories that illuminate core conflicts and relationship issues.

The core conflictual relationship theme (CCRT) method can be used as an organizing framework to help reveal the core conflict that forms the basis for all of the patient's relationships. By drawing on the above descriptions of Flora's interactions with both the therapist and her father, Flora's core conflict can be understood as follows: The patient wishes (W) to be praised by the therapist. She perceives the therapist's response (R_O) as critical and becomes silent and withdrawn (R_S). Similarly, the patient wished (W) to be admired by her father. When he responded with criticism (R_O), she felt humiliated and withdrew (R_S). Identifying the core conflict early in treatment provides a central focus for the work of therapy and enhances the therapeutic alliance.

In supportive and cognitive-behavioral psychotherapies, the connection between transference reactions and the past is generally not explored; rather, transference reactions are understood as examples of the patient's behavior with current figures in his or her life. In these approaches, it is preferable to remain focused on the patient-therapist relationship. However, if the patient makes a link to the past, the therapist should be ready to listen and explore, emphasizing a cognitive rather than an affective approach. For individuals in the middle of the psychotherapy continuum, it may be appropriate to introduce and explore linkages between transference reactions and the past later in therapy, after a positive therapeutic relationship has been established.

Many of the innovators of short-term dynamic psychotherapy advocated early and frequent interpretation of the transference (Davanloo 1980; Malan 1976; Sifneos 1979). Malan (1976) reported that therapists' use of transference interpretations linked to parental figures correlated with patient improvement. However, other investigators were unable to replicate these findings (Marziali 1984; Piper et al. 1986). Piper and colleagues (1991) subsequently reported a negative correlation between frequent transference interpretations and favorable outcome in patients with a high quality of object relations. This finding implies that negative effects can ensue from excessive use of transference interpretations, a practice Gill (1982) cautioned against. Another possible explanation is that negative treatment effects consisting of sustained patient anger toward the therapist, poor alliance, or significant resistance may induce therapists to respond with increased transference interpretations in an attempt to repair the misalliance.

Therapists evoke transference reactions by what they say and how they say it. These reactions reveal the patient's style of responding and/or their personality characteristics. In the trial therapy of Derrick described in Chapter 3, the therapist asked about the patient's feelings toward an individual who was late and disappointed him. Derrick responded defensively, and the therapist addressed his defensive behavior. Confrontation of Derrick's defenses evoked Derrick's characteristic way of responding to a woman. He experienced the female therapist as critical and became angry, but was unable to express this anger directly.

Therapist errors invariably occur and play a vital role in psychotherapy. These mistakes may or may not be within the therapist's awareness. However, listening to material with attention to hidden meanings and allusions to the therapeutic relationship can be helpful in alerting therapists to their errors. In the example given earlier of Flora, who told her therapist that she had recently been confiding more in her sisters, the therapist asked the patient if she were having trouble confiding in him. Flora became silent, and the therapist realized that something was wrong. Exploration revealed that the patient felt criticized. This provided the therapist with an opportunity to repair the misalliance. In this example, the therapist may have jumped to an erroneous conclusion by assuming that Flora's confiding in her sisters meant that she was unable to confide in him. An alternative explanation might be that her improved ability to confide in her sisters was related to her positive relationship with the therapist. Therefore, a more open-ended question— such as "What are your thoughts about confiding more in your sisters lately?"— might not have produced a misalliance.

When therapist errors occur, they should be acknowledged. Not to do so is confusing to the patient because it distorts what really has transpired. This is especially true if the therapist explores the error and directly or indirectly blames the patient, is dismissive, or shrugs it off as transference.

> A therapist became drowsy and failed to hear what the patient was saying. When confronted by the patient, the therapist said: "You were repeating something you have said many times, so I tuned out, the way others do with you."

This therapist needs to acknowledge his drowsiness to avoid confusing the patient by making excuses and distorting reality. A simple apology is called for in this situation. The interpretation offered is defensive and blames the patient for evoking drowsiness in the therapist. The countertransference issues raised in this example will be discussed in the following section.

Countertransference

Classically, countertransference is the therapist's transference to the patient (Greenson 1967). It includes behaviors, feelings, thoughts, wishes, attitudes, and conflicts derived from the therapist's past and displaced onto the patient. A broader definition of countertransference includes the real relationship, consisting of reactions most people would have to the patient determined by moment-to-moment interactions in the therapeutic relationship. The therapist's countertransference reactions can lead him or her to misunderstand the patient and can result in inappropriate behavior toward the patient. Countertransference reactions can also be a powerful tool for understanding and empathizing with the patient.

Countertransference and transference reactions may be more or less weighted by both past and present. Therefore, all interactions within the therapeutic relationship are based on a combination of the real relationship and the transference/countertransference configuration.

The following is an example of classical countertransference.

> A female therapist was treating a male patient several years younger than herself who spoke about being nasty to and making fun of his sister at a family party. As the patient related this story, the therapist became increasingly uneasy and began to question the patient in a prosecutorial manner. When the patient appeared wounded, the therapist realized that her questions were harsh. Later, when reflecting on the session, the therapist recognized that her behavior was derived from conflicts with a younger brother who behaved in a similar manner.

In this example, the therapist's past experiences with her brother strongly influenced her inappropriate response to the patient. Undoubtedly the patient's story had meaning in the present context of the patient-therapist relationship, but the past experience of the therapist was a more important factor.

An example of countertransference derived more from the real or current situation follows.

> A patient in his late 30s asked his therapist to add additional sessions to the insurance form so that he would not be responsible for the copayment. The therapist viewed this request negatively, felt put on the spot, and indicated that he could not comply.

Were this therapist's feeling and response related to a past experience? Certainly, but the reality aspects of this encounter appear to outweigh past influences.

Use of the Countertransference

These examples of countertransference illustrate problems in the patient-therapist relationship. At the same time, however, countertransference problems present opportunities for greater understanding of the patient and the therapeutic relationship. To accomplish this, therapists must monitor their own feelings and reactions toward their patients.

The use of empathy is important in facilitating, impeding, or distorting countertransference awareness. Empathy can be defined as "feeling oneself into" something or somebody (Wolf 1983, p. 309). Therefore, empathy is a method of gathering data about the mental life of another person. The ability to empathize by accurately sensing and understanding what a patient is experiencing will enable the therapist to attend to countertransference reactions.

The examples provided illustrate how countertransference reactions can be used therapeutically. If the therapist who had conflicts with her brother had monitored her reaction to the patient's story, realized that her reaction to the patient was based on her own experience, and been able to be empathic toward the patient, she might have been able to offer a more therapeutic response. She could have said, "I wonder what you were experiencing as you made fun of your sister? As you related the story, I sensed that you did not really feel comfortable telling me what you did." In a more supportive or cognitive psychotherapy, the therapist could have asked the patient for thoughts instead of feelings or experiences.

In the second example, the therapist felt put on the spot when asked to falsify records. This was a reaction to the reality of what the patient was requesting, the patient's transference wishes, and the therapist's own reality and neurotic needs. Self-reflection enabled the therapist to use his countertransference reactions to explore the meaning of the patient's request. This therapist should ask himself, "What is motivating this patient's request, and what is it about his request that evokes these feelings in me?" In this case, possible answers include "the patient is needy and wants more help from me," "the patient is asking me to break the law, which makes me feel uncomfortable and prevents me from exploring his request," and "the patient is trying to test me."

The Real Relationship

The real relationship underlies all psychotherapy. It exists in the here and now of the therapeutic interaction between patient and therapist, encompassing a genuine mutual liking for each other that is authentic, trusting, and realistic without the distortions that are characteristic of transference (Greenson 1967, 1971). The real relationship includes the patient's hopes and aspirations for help, care, understanding, and love, as well as the everyday interactions that take place on a social level between individuals. In addition, "moments of implicit relational knowing" (Stern et al. (1998, p. 903) take place between patient and therapist that are outside conscious verbal experience. In these moments, an "authentic person-to-person connection...

with the therapist [occurs] that alters the relationship...and thereby the patient's sense of himself" (p. 904). As a result, a change is created in the intersubjective relationship for both patient and therapist.

As discussed earlier, the real relationship and the transference may not be separable. A person's behavior and attitudes toward others have to do with both past and present, as the following example illustrates.

> A new patient who was unemployed was disappointed at the end of the initial session when the therapist did not offer to get him a job. What the patient wanted from the therapist was real, because he needed a job, but at the same time it was related to the patient's wish to have others take care of him as his mother did.

In expressive psychotherapy, the real relationship and the transference both play central roles. In supportive and cognitive-behavioral psychotherapies, the real relationship is paramount and transference issues are minimized. At the same time, the therapist is mindful of the transference but generally does not interpret it. At the middle of the continuum, where most therapies are conducted, the work of therapy is primarily on the real relationship. Transference interpretations can at times be useful, but they should not play a major role in treatment at this point on the continuum.

The Therapeutic Alliance

The therapeutic alliance is part of the real relationship. According to Zetzel (1956, 1966), an alliance is necessary to support the work of psychotherapy. She believed that the capacity to form an alliance is based on an individual's early developmental experiences with the primary caretaker. In the absence of this capacity, the task of the therapist, early in treatment, is to provide a supportive relationship to foster development of a therapeutic alliance.

Greenson (1967) emphasized the collaborative nature of the alliance, in which patient and therapist work together to promote therapeutic change. Bordin (1979) operationalized the therapeutic alliance concept as the degree of agreement between patient and therapist concerning the tasks and goals of psychotherapy and the quality of the bond between them. He conceptualized the alliance as evolving and changing as the result of a dynamic interactive process occurring between patient and therapist. The tasks and goals of therapy are subject to change as a result of the ongoing give-and-take relationship in the patient-therapist dyad.

Gaston (1990), building on Bordin's work, elaborated four dimensions of the alliance: 1) the patient's affective bond to the therapist and commitment to therapy, 2) the patient's capacity to work purposefully in therapy, 3) the therapist's empathic understanding and involvement, and 4) the agreement of patient and therapist on the tasks and goals of therapy. Gaston's major additions are the therapist's empathic understanding, which serves to deepen the bond dimension, and the patient's capacity to work in therapy, as stressed by Greenson.

Establishing a positive therapeutic alliance is essential for most psychotherapies, but especially brief psychotherapy (Bordin 1979). The alliance or therapeutic relationship is central to most treatments and has been identified as one of the ingredients shared by nearly all forms of psychotherapy (see Chapters 5 and 10 for a discussion of these common factors). Outcome research has led to the idea that the common factors may be critical change agents in most psychotherapies (Butler and Strupp 1986; Luborsky et al. 1993). In some psychotherapies the alliance may be the change agent in and of itself, whereas in other treatments the alliance may act as a background for therapeutic interventions (Westerman et al. 1995). A growing body of evidence supports the idea that the quality of the therapeutic alliance is the best predictor of outcome in brief psychotherapy (Gaston 1990; Horvath and Symonds 1991). This has been found to be true for many different types of therapy, including dynamic, experiential, cognitive-behavioral, and group psychotherapy (L. S. Greenberg et al. 1993; Luborsky 1976; MacKenzie 1998; Muran and Ventur 1995). If the alliance becomes problematic, it is critical that it be repaired quickly, because time is of the essence.

Alliance Ruptures

The stability of the therapeutic alliance appears to be related to the psychotherapy continuum. The alliance tends to be more stable on the supportive side of the continuum than on the expressive end, because it is not threatened by challenging confrontations or interpretations, which may heighten patient anxiety (Hellerstein et al. 1998). Expressive therapy may produce more ruptures in the alliance because of its use of challenging techniques. In the middle of the continuum, the potential for disruption of the alliance is related to how the therapist balances the use of supportive and expressive interventions.

Patients vary in their capacity to establish a positive alliance with a therapist. Those on the left side of the psychopathology–psychological structure continuum, with structural deficits, especially in object relations, may have problems developing a positive relationship with the therapist. The inability to develop "basic trust" (Erikson 1950) interferes with the establishment of a therapeutic bond. With these patients, a major therapeutic task, especially early in treatment, is building a trusting relationship.

Another group of patients, those more in the middle of the psychopathology–psychological structure continuum (e.g., individuals with personality disorders), often have significant interpersonal problems. There is evidence to indicate that hostile–dominant problems are negatively related, and overly friendly–submissive problems positively related, to the development of the alliance (L.M. Horowitz et al. 1993; Muran et al. 1994; A. Winston et al. 1994a) (see Chapter 10 for a discussion of the terms *hostile–dominant* and *friendly–submissive*).

Breaks in the alliance are not unusual. In fact, misunderstandings between therapist and patient occur for a number of reasons. Over the course of psychotherapy, the patient may at various times experience the therapist as critical, insensitive, distant, withholding, untrustworthy, intrusive, unempathic, and so on, which will contribute to a misalliance. One of the most effective ways of involving the patient in the treatment process is to listen to what the patient is conveying. If the therapist can understand the patient's manifest and latent communications, therapist recognition of a misalliance will be facilitated.

Therapists vary in their ability to establish and maintain a therapeutic alliance. Warmth, respectfulness, genuineness, and empathy are essential therapist qualities for developing and maintaining a therapeutic bond (Lewis 1978). Some clinicians are naturally gifted in this area, while others can be educated to develop these qualities. This should be a major focus in the training and supervision of therapists. The following is an example of a problem in this area.

> A patient in supportive psychotherapy, who regularly kept appointments, failed to appear at a session. The therapist did not attempt to contact the patient. In the next session, the patient began by angrily asking the therapist why there had been no attempt to contact her. The patient explained that she had been ill and taken to the hospital.

In any psychotherapy, but particularly supportive treatment, the patient should have been called. Doing so would have conveyed respect for and interest in the patient.

Educating patients about the tasks and goals of psychotherapy sets the stage for the collaborative nature of the work that lies ahead. The therapist should be explicit about how the therapy works. For example, in expressive psychotherapy, the therapist should explain the exploratory process, how it can lead to understanding problems, enabling patients to make changes in their lives. Goals should be mutually agreed upon, realistic, and open to negotiation as therapy proceeds (see Chapter 5 for a discussion of tasks and goals).

Even after an alliance is established, breaks or ruptures can occur. Therapist contributions to breaches in the alliance include technical errors, countertransference issues, lack of empathy at certain times, inflexibility, and so on. Technical errors commonly occur and usually do not produce a misalliance. Often, patients simply correct the therapist, recognizing that therapists, like everyone else, make mistakes. However, at times an error will be disruptive. An example of a technical error that can be problematic is the use of challenging interventions with a patient in supportive therapy. Similarly, employing excessive supportive techniques with a high-functioning patient can interfere with autonomy and produce a misalliance.

Inflexibility can be a major impediment to treatment. A patient who began supportive-expressive psychotherapy with great reluctance immediately asked for changes in appointment times. The therapist was unwilling to be flexible, and the patient became furious and left treatment. A more flexible therapist, recognizing the patient's ambivalence toward treatment, would have accommodated the patient and then been in a position to explore her need to change appointments. This patient was in the habit of testing others to see if they would accede to her requests. When someone disappointed her, she would discard them as she discarded the therapist.

Although there is little evidence in the research literature on the effect of the therapist's personality on the alliance, most practitioners would agree that it plays a significant role. Henry et al. (1990) reported evidence indicating that therapists with self-hostile introjects (i.e., hostile self-concept) engaged in more interpersonal hostility and complex communications during the course of therapy.

While ruptures in the alliance can be disruptive and problematic, they can also present opportunities for patient interpersonal growth and change. We need to improve our understanding of breaches in the alliance and how to repair them. This may help with patients who do poorly in psychotherapy. Foreman and Marmar (1985) examined patients with poor therapeutic alliances and found that confrontation of defensive behavior led to improved therapeutic alliance and outcome, whereas in unimproved patients, defenses were not addressed. B. Winston and colleagues (1994) found that a greater frequency of addressing defensive behavior correlated with decreased defensiveness and a positive outcome at termination in brief dynamic psychotherapy.

Ryle (1979) described the various types of impasses occurring in the alliance as snags, traps, or dilemmas. In a controlled/controlling dilemma, for example, the patient feels either helplessly submissive or excessively powerful with another individual. In a distance/closeness dilemma, the patient feels excessively isolated or at risk from being too close. M. Horowitz and Marmar (1985) suggested that when the therapist attempts to interpret or explore both horns of the dilemma with a "difficult" patient (e.g., a patient with a severe personality disorder), the most likely outcome is a misalliance. In such an event, they recommend an empathic holding approach, as suggested by Winnicott (1965).

The process of repairing ruptures in the therapeutic alliance is gradually being delineated (Safran et al. 1990, 1994; A. Winston and Muran 1996). A model is being developed that has the potential to provide clinicians with information about the dynamic interactional sequences associated with improvement in the therapeutic alliance. Two types of ruptures or misalliances have been described: confrontation and withdrawal (Safran and Muran 1998). In a confrontational type of misalliance, the patient expresses anger or dissatisfaction with the therapist or the therapy. For example, a patient confronts his therapist by saying, "What am I getting in this treatment? I knew most of what you've said before I came." In a withdrawal rupture, the patient disengages from the therapist: "I almost didn't come today. I have nothing to talk about." Regardless of where the patient is on the psychopathology–psychological structure continuum, such expressions must be explored. Patients who are able to be direct (i.e., those who are less defensive) will express their underlying wish, need, or feeling. It will be the therapist's task to encourage an open exploration of these wishes, needs, or feelings. Central to this process is the therapist's ability to explore his or her own contribution to the misalliance nondefensively. Through this process, patients develop the ability to express their dissatisfactions clearly and directly, while the therapist acknowledges this positive behavior.

When patients are more defensive, exploration of misalliances will be blocked. Two types of blocks have been described (Safran and Muran 1998). The first consists of thoughts, beliefs, and expectations about the therapist or others. Inherent in the patient's belief system is the idea that others will react in a negative manner if the patient expresses his or her true thoughts, wishes, or beliefs. The negative response anticipated from the other may be inattention, criticism, or retaliation. The following vignette illustrates this type of block.

> A man told his therapist that he wanted to take some time off from treatment because of his busy schedule. Underlying this statement was the patient's dissatisfaction with the therapist for not being helpful enough. The

patient was unable to be direct with the therapist because he feared that the therapist would be critical and retaliate.

The second type of block is based on the patient's self-critical or self-doubting processes:

> A patient missed a session following the therapist's vacation. Exploration revealed that a crisis had occurred during the therapist's absence. However, when the therapist tried to elicit the patient's thoughts and feelings about the therapist's absence, the patient replied, "You're entitled to a vacation; I can't expect you to be around for me." Her belief was that she was unworthy of concern or attention.

When a block interferes with exploration of a misalliance, the therapist should first address the patient's avoidance and then explore the patient's belief system or defensive behavior causing the block. Such exploration facilitates the expression of the underlying wish, need, or feeling that led to the misalliance.

Repair of misalliances is one of the most crucial aspects of psychotherapy. Such repair provides the patient with a "corrective emotional experience"— a departure from the past that constitutes a new and positive interaction with another, more benign person (Alexander and French 1946). In addition, a reparative experience occurs when the therapist is able to acknowledge his or her errors and contribution to the alliance rupture. In the second example above, the alliance was repaired when the therapist acknowledged the patient's wish to have her available during the crisis and expressed regret for being away.

The end point in the repair of alliance ruptures is the free expression of the patient's feelings (and wishes) in a direct and clear manner to the therapist, who in turn validates and confirms the patient's communication. The same type of rupture may occur again and will need to be worked through in a similar manner. The misalliance repair cycle presents the clinician with a powerful therapeutic opportunity when approached nondefensively. No one enjoys being the object of negative feelings or criticism, and many therapists naturally avoid their exploration. Both experienced and beginning therapists need to exercise vigilance to maintain the therapeutic relationship by monitoring their countertransference reactions.

5

Essential Elements and Interventions

Knowledge of the essential elements and interventions of brief treatment is vital to sound clinical practice. These essential ingredients are drawn from the principles of brief psychotherapy and provide the structure for its interventions. Technical interventions are derived from expressive, supportive, and cognitive-behavioral psychotherapies. The clinician, as a prerequisite to practice, should have an understanding of the essentials of brief treatment, which consist of 1) a time limit, 2) a maintained focus, 3) a high activity level on the part of the therapist, 4) explicit goals, 5) patient motivation, and 6) a positive therapeutic relationship. As the indispensable ingredient of psychotherapy, the patient-therapist relationship has been accorded its own chapter (see Chapter 4). We begin with a discussion of the essential ingredients of brief treatment, and follow this with an explication of the interventions.

Essential Elements

Time Limit

Time-limited psychotherapy creates an atmosphere in which both patient and therapist understand that time is of the essence. It exerts pressure so that both participants work hard and stay focused to achieve the desired goals (Alexander and French 1946; Mann 1973). Time limits vary from treatment to treatment. Treatments are generally flexible in terms of the number of sessions, with most falling in the 15- to 30-session range. Some authors have advocated a fixed number of sessions, such as Mann (1973), who adhered to a 12-session treatment, while Davanloo (1980) held to an upper limit of 40 sessions. Establishing a time limit sets the stage for patient and therapist to explore separation and loss in the therapeutic relationship. As a result, separation and loss can first be worked through in the therapeutic relationship and then be connected to important people in the patient's life.

Outcome research has demonstrated the efficacy of brief psychotherapy (Crits-Christoph 1992; Piper et al. 1991; A. Winston et al. 1994a). There is little evidence indicating superiority of either short- or long-term treatment. Indeed, Howard et al. (1986) showed that patient improvement takes place early in treatment and that 75% of patients have improved by the 26th session (see Chapter 10 for a discussion of research issues).

Maintenance of Focus

A generally accepted principle of brief psychotherapy is maintenance of focus by the therapist (Beck et al. 1979; Davanloo 1980; Malan 1976; Sabin 1981; Sifneos 1972). Essentially, if the therapist maintains a focus, drift into secondary issues is minimized and the patient's defensive behavior is highlighted. The therapist needs to be active and refocus when the patient strays from the issue at hand. Defensive behavior characteristically is used by patients to avoid painful affects, thoughts, and memories. Accordingly, therapists need to confront, clarify, interpret, educate, and set session agendas and homework assignments, so that patients come to understand their patterns of behavior and how they avoid focusing on painful material. Davanloo (1980) used the term *holding* to describe the intensive process of focusing that he employed with highly resistant patients. In a study of patients with personality disorders, B. Winston et al. (1994) found that outcome in brief dynamic psychotherapy was enhanced by a greater frequency of addressing defensive behavior. However, the techniques of confronting defenses and refocusing patients on painful affects are generally avoided in supportive psychotherapy.

High Activity Level of Therapist

In brief psychotherapy, a high level of activity is required of the therapist. The time limit will not allow the therapist to sit back and wait for issues to unfold. The clinician must actively engage the patient so that work on behavior change is possible. In brief integrated therapy, therapists apply techniques based on the patient's position on the psychological structure/ psychotherapy continuum. On the expressive side, interventions aim at uncovering underlying wishes, needs, and feelings. The techniques used include confronting and clarifying defenses, addressing automatic thoughts, offering interpretations, and holding the patient to the focus. On the supportive side of the continuum, interventions are used to reduce anxiety, enhance self-esteem, and improve ego functioning and adaptation. Techniques include advice giving, praise, rehearsal, reframing, and cognitive restructuring. The therapeutic alliance should be actively monitored at all times so that a poor alliance can be quickly repaired. Unlike long-term therapy, brief psychotherapy will generally fail if a breach in the alliance lasts more than a few sessions (Samstag et al. 1998).

Explicit Goals

Setting goals during the initial evaluation in brief psychotherapy is mandatory, not optional. An agreement about the objectives of treatment should be achieved within the first one or two meetings. Although most psychotherapists have general ideas about how to proceed and what might be accomplished in treatment, treatment goals often are not discussed. We believe that goals should be explicit in all forms of psychotherapy, and especially brief psychotherapy.

Because of the pressure of time, the therapist needs to be cognizant of both immediate objectives for each session and overall goals for treatment. An immediate in-session objective may be to develop a mutually agreed-upon plan for a job interview, while a long-term goal might be to promote job stability.

Clearly outlined aims help motivate patients and promote the therapeutic alliance as both patient and therapist work toward a common end. Connecting problem areas to the goals of treatment increases patients' motivation to change and promotes therapeutic clarity. Specified goals provide a requisite focus for both patient and therapist. With the end points of treatment in mind, the therapist can hold the patient to the essential issues, even when both may be tempted to take a detour, thus lengthening the therapeutic process.

How extensive can goals be? Is it possible to alter personality patterns and achieve so-called structural change in a short period of time? There is evidence from a number of studies (Piper et al. 1991; Rosenthal et al. 1999; A. Winston et al. 1994a; B. Winston et al. 1994) that maladaptive character patterns, including defenses, can indeed change significantly over the course of brief treatment. Rosenthal et al. (1999) demonstrated significant change in interpersonal functioning in patients with personality disorders treated with brief supportive psychotherapy.

Traditionally we think of goals as accomplishments achieved at the end of treatment. However, it may be more useful to think of a goal as ranging from immediate to ultimate (Parloff 1967). An *immediate* in-session goal would be to clarify an interpersonal distortion, whereas an *ultimate* goal might be to enable the patient to achieve a meaningful interpersonal relationship.

The following vignettes illustrate immediate and ultimate goals.

> Rose is a 48-year-old divorced woman who idealizes her ex-husband despite his many failings. He had numerous extramarital affairs and embezzled large amounts of money from his boss, leaving Rose to make reparations. In an early session, Rose spoke glowingly about her ex-husband and his charismatic style of behavior. The therapist highlighted Rose's dysfunctional thinking by pointing out that her husband had left her with no financial support and the responsibility for his debts. The immediate goal was to clarify the patient's distorted view of her ex-husband. Rose had developed a long-term relationship with another man who was caring, honest, and admiring of her, yet she was unwilling to make a commitment to him. The ultimate goal was to enable Rose to have a satisfying and close relationship with this man.

> Martin, a 42-year-old man with troubling obsessions and compulsions, as well as interpersonal problems with his children, was opposed to cognitive-behavioral treatment because it had failed in the past; he was also hesitant to try medication. An immediate objective would be to help Art accept medication or cognitive-behavioral treatment, while the ultimate goals would be the amelioration of his obsessive-compulsive symptoms and an improvement in his relationship with his children.

Treatment goals should always be discussed and formulated with the patient. The therapist must listen carefully to determine areas of difficulty in the patient's life and develop an understanding of the patient's problems, wishes, and needs. The use of structured and semistructured questionnaires can be helpful in formulating treatment goals. Questionnaires enable patients to think about their problems in a concrete and organized manner and help to minimize denial. A useful tool is the outlining of target complaints (TCs) (Battle et al. 1966) with the patient. The TC approach requires the patient and therapist to list and rate the patient's major problems. Generally, the complaints are limited to three major issues and are rated on a scale of

1 to 13, with 13 being the most severe. TCs can lead to clear goals that are readily accessible to both patient and therapist.

The example below illustrates the use of target complaints.

> Bob, a 30-year-old man, presented for treatment with the following complaints: 1) I don't have a satisfying relationship with a woman, 2) I am too financially dependent on my father, and 3) I have not been successful in my work. The patient rated these problems as very troubling on the 1–13 scale: 11, 10, and 11, respectively. The therapist felt that Bob's assessments were accurate. He and the patient reframed the target complaints into treatment goals—for example, the second goal became Bob's financial independence from his father.

Establishing clearly articulated goals is helpful in maintaining a therapeutic focus in brief therapy. Reciprocally, maintenance of focus aids the therapeutic dyad in reaching the stated therapeutic goals.

A basic rule of treatment is that the goals of therapy should generally be the patient's. In the event of disagreement on goals, the therapist enters into an exploration of the problem, as illustrated below.

> Gail, a 63-year-old widow, came into treatment with two clearly defined goals: 1) to have the courage to sell her house and move to an apartment and 2) to find a satisfying job. The therapist felt that these goals were too limited and suggested an open-ended treatment so that Gail could accomplish more.

If a therapist-patient disagreement regarding treatment goals is not quickly resolved, an alliance rupture will ensue.

The importance of setting realistic goals with the patient cannot be overemphasized, particularly with patients who have severe psychopathology, as in the following example.

> Doris is a 41-year-old woman with major depressive disorder, significant dependency on others, and separation problems. When faced with difficult situations, she uses fantasy rather than confronting the painful realities of her life. Her husband is physically brutal, controlling, and verbally abusive to Doris and their daughter. Doris fantasized that his behavior would change and that her marriage would become ideal. However, her husband refused to get help for himself or to participate in Doris' treatment. A more realistic goal for Doris might be to acknowledge the impasse with her husband and consider a separation. The therapist used explanation to help Doris to understand how she slipped into fantasy to avoid the painful reality of her husband's behavior.

Explanation helps to heighten patients' awareness of the issues they are struggling with and to promote understanding. Although many therapists rely heavily on the use of explanation throughout the course of treatment, this tool is particularly valuable when mapping out realistic goals with patients.

Some patients enter treatment with goals based on magical wishes, as illustrated below.

> Ed, a 53-year-old unemployed appliance repairman, expected the therapist to magically change what was most troubling in his life at the moment. In the first session, the therapist learned that Ed was a dependent, passive man who expected others to look after him. Toward the end of the evaluation, Ed became downhearted and stated that he was disappointed. He went on to explain that he had thought that the therapist would pick up the telephone, call a friend, and get him a job.

This vignette highlights a patient's unrealistic fantasy based on a dysfunctional way of thinking. By clarifying the patient's wish, a more realistic goal can be negotiated with the patient so that a plan can be devised to help him get back to work. Later, the patient's dysfunctional thinking (schema-based) should be addressed so that he can learn to behave in a more active manner.

It should be noted that goals can be renegotiated as treatment proceeds. Many patients enter treatment requesting help with conditions such as panic attacks or depression.

> Peter, a 35-year-old man who had been married for 5 years, came into treatment with both panic and dysthymic disorders. He was treated with medication and brief integrated psychotherapy and improved within 5 weeks. During the sixth session, Peter told the therapist that he now wanted help so that he could be more assertive, especially at work. Patient and therapist agreed to work on this problem using assertiveness training.

Patient Motivation

Patient motivation is an important factor in psychotherapy and its outcome. When patients are highly motivated to work on what is problematic in their lives, therapy is facilitated. Highly motivated patients are generally less resistant and establish a therapeutic alliance more readily. Sifneos (1972) believed that motivation to change predicted a successful outcome. He outlined the following criteria for assessing patient motivation: 1) recognition on the patient's part that the symptoms are psychological; 2) introspective ability accompanied by an honest and truthful account of emotional difficulties; 3) willingness to participate actively in treatment and to change, explore, experiment, and make reasonable sacrifices; and 4) curiosity and willingness to understand oneself and to have realistic expectations about psychotherapy.

Many patients are not highly motivated, especially those who seek treatment at the urging of others. However, even these patients can be motivated by a therapeutic experience within the initial evaluation (Davanloo 1980). The therapeutic experience helps to promote interest and curiosity about oneself. As the patient becomes interested in learning about his or her behaviors and problems, the idea that change is possible begins to develop. With the sense that change can take place, hope is awakened within the patient. In more expressive psychotherapy, the patient's belief in the possibility of change is further enhanced by understanding the negative impact of maladaptive behavior and thoughts. In more supportive psychotherapy, the belief in the possibility of change is augmented by the therapist's listening, conveying interest and understanding, and framing the problems in terms of self-esteem regulation and everyday functioning in life. Finally, a therapeutic experience helps to promote a positive therapeutic relationship, which is a motivating force for the patient.

Techniques for providing a therapeutic experience may include giving advice or praise, explaining, interpreting, clarifying and/or confronting defensive behavior, using motivational interventions, and wrapping up or summarizing key elements from the session. The techniques employed will depend on the patient's location on the psychopathology–psychological structure continuum. A full description of psychotherapy techniques appears later in this chapter.

Motivational interventions are expressed as either questions or statements by the therapist. They set the stage for a dialogue between patient and therapist to explore the reasons for and consequences of lack of motivation. They are explicit in stating that painful aspects of the patient's life will remain the same unless defensive behavior changes. The following vignettes illustrate the use of motivational interventions.

> In an evaluation session using expressive trial therapy, a patient persistently avoided painful affects when confronted by the therapist. The therapist posed the following motivational question: "If you continue to avoid your feelings here with me, how will we understand what's going on within you?"

> In another evaluation interview using supportive trial therapy, a patient expressed feelings of shame about her problem and was reluctant to tell the

therapist what was troubling her. She feared that the therapist would find her problem to be "stupid and trivial." Even after an exploration of her expectations regarding the therapist, she continued to avoid describing the problem that had brought her to treatment. The therapist finally said, "I understand that your judgment of my response is preventing you from being direct with me, but if we can't examine the problem together, how can I be of help to you?"

Patient Selection, Assessment, and Case Formulation

Patient selection, assessment, and case formulation are key elements in brief integrated psychotherapy. A thorough discussion of these important ingredients was presented in Chapter 3.

Interventions

Many technical interventions are available to the therapist. They are drawn from cognitive-behavioral, interpersonal, and psychoanalytic models. How to choose an appropriate approach is a problem for many clinicians, whether they are just beginning or more experienced. Technique is dependent on the clinician's assessment of the patient and the patient's location on the psychopathology–psychological structure continuum. That location, in turn, will help determine where the patient fits on the psychotherapy continuum and will aid in determining the best approach to the patient (see Chapter 3).

A patient whose psychological structure is relatively intact will be on the expressive side of the psychotherapy continuum, and the treatment approach will be primarily based on the conflict model (see Chapter 2). The patient whose psychological structure is less intact will be on the supportive side of the psychotherapy continuum. In actual clinical practice, many patients are located at the center of the psychological structure/psychotherapy continua and are best treated with an integrated approach that combines supportive, expressive, and cognitive-behavioral techniques.

Therapeutic measures are most effective in the presence of a positive therapeutic relationship. The therapeutic alliance requires constant monitoring during psychotherapy, especially during the course of brief psychotherapy. In the presence of a poor alliance, most interventions will fail unless directed at repairing the misalliance.

One of the best ways to maintain an alliance is to be a good listener. Generally, therapists need to listen to what patients say on many different levels, both conscious and unconscious, so that they develop an understanding of what patients mean. A concept that helps direct therapists' attention to the underlying meaning of patients' communications is the "adaptive context" (Langs 1978). We have found the concept to be clinically useful when it is broadened to include the various dynamic forces in operation as the patient enters the therapist's office and begins the session. Often, the patient's opening statements herald the content of the session and provide the adaptive context. If the therapist is listening carefully, he or she may be rewarded with an understanding of the adaptive context and as a result be prepared for what may unfold (see clinical examples in Cases 2, 3, and 4 in Chapters 7, 8, and 9).

The interventions described below are divided into supportive, cognitive-behavioral, and expressive categories to present them in as clear a manner as possible. In actual practice, however, these different techniques are often combined, especially in an integrated approach. At the end of this chapter, we will compare and contrast dynamic/interpersonal with cognitive-behavioral therapy. In addition, we will focus on the important concept and technique of transitioning among supportive, cognitive-behavioral, and expressive interventions.

Supportive Techniques

Supportive psychotherapy depends on clearly defined techniques designed to achieve the goal of maintaining or improving the patient's self-esteem, ego functioning, and adaptation to the environment (Pinsker et al. 1991). In supportive treatment, the objectives include reduction of anxiety, promotion of stability, and relief of symptoms. These goals are accomplished primarily by working in the here and now rather than in the past. The therapeutic relationship becomes a focus in a real as opposed to a transferential manner (see Chapter 4). Generally, resistance is not addressed, and defenses are strengthened and supported. However, if a defense is maladaptive, it should be addressed. For instance, an individual who believes that others think that he is a child molester and that they intend to hurt him needs help with these projections, which are of a paranoid type.

Style of Communication

The style of supportive psychotherapy is usually conversational. Silences are generally to be avoided, because they tend to raise the individual's level of anxiety. There should be a give-and-take exchange, and challenging questions—especially those that the patient may find difficult to answer—should not be asked. Questions beginning with "Why" should be avoided, since they can increase anxiety and threaten self-esteem.

Clarification, Confrontation, and Interpretation

Clarification is central to the style of communication between patient and therapist. In our approach, it is the most frequently used intervention. Clarification consists of a restatement and summary of what the patient has told the therapist without elaboration or inference. Clarification frames a communication so that both parties agree on what is being discussed. Summarizing and restating help organize the patient's thinking and provide structure. They demonstrate that the therapist is listening and attending to what the patient is saying. In the example below, a clarification is provided:

> Patient: Yesterday a co-worker asked me a lot of questions. I tried to continue working, but I couldn't.

> Therapist: So your co-worker's questions interfered with your work despite your efforts.

This clarification framed the patient's communication so that it could be explored.

Confrontation addresses a patient's defensive behavior. In supportive psychotherapy, confrontations generally should be empathically framed. They are used to address maladaptive defenses; adaptive defenses are encouraged. Confrontation in a supportive mode is illustrated below:

> Patient: I walked into a room and there were lots of people, and a lot of strangers. They weren't talking about anything interesting, so I left.

> Therapist: Walking into a room with strangers is hard for you, so you left, but I wonder if thinking that they weren't talking about anything interesting is your way of avoiding a difficult situation.

Here, the therapist's empathic clarification is followed by a confrontation.

An interpretation is an explanation that brings meaning to the patient's behavior or thinking. Generally, it makes the individual aware of something that was not previously conscious. An interpretation can link thoughts, feelings, and behaviors toward people in the patient's current life to people from the past and/or to the therapist. In supportive psychotherapy, interpretation is generally more limited in scope. Present rather than past relationships are emphasized; affects and impulses are rarely interpreted. Incomplete or inexact interpretations (Glover 1931) offer explanations that are plausible and help the patient make sense of his or her experience but do not contain material that might disturb the patient. For example, a fragile patient who is tormented by unacceptable homosexual thoughts whenever he gets close to a woman might be offered the following inexact interpretation:

> Therapist: Whenever you begin to establish a long-sought-for relationship with a woman, you begin to worry about sexual intimacy and protect yourself against these worries by having homosexual thoughts about men.

In expressive psychotherapy, defenses are more often challenged so that patients are encouraged to become aware of their characteristic styles of behavior and motivation. For example, passivity generally is confronted in expressive psychotherapy, whereas in supportive psychotherapy the patient is encouraged to think about choices or options that can be activating and lead to desired goals.

Praise, Reassurance, Encouragement, and Advice

Praise, reassurance, and encouragement are useful techniques for promoting patient self-esteem. The therapist should be genuine when using these techniques (Lewis 1978). Patients quickly pick up on comments that are patronizing or gratuitous and may feel misunderstood. Inauthenticity can seriously undermine the therapeutic relationship. Praise, when offered, should be reality based. A patient who attends a lecture as part of a psychotherapy homework assignment involving socialization can be realistically praised—for example, "It's terrific that you got yourself to go!"

Words spoken in an attempt to reassure a patient must not be empty or without basis. Many patients ask their therapist if they will get better. A response of "Yes, you will get better" may be misleading and false. A more appropriate response would be "Most people with your condition improve."

It is useful to think about encouragement as a form of coaching. In supportive psychotherapy, coaching frequently is used to help patients try new approaches to problems and engage in different behaviors and activities (Pinsker 1998). The activities can be social, recreational, educational, or vocational, as illustrated below.

> A patient complained that she was inept because she was unable to write a cover letter for a job application. The therapist said, "Let's see what we can do now to help you get started."

Advice should be based on the therapist's knowledge and expertise in the field of psychotherapy. In contrast to the more abstinent therapeutic stance employed in expressive psychotherapy, the therapist conducting supportive therapy should feel comfortable being direct and taking an active role with patients.

> A patient called his therapist and reported that he couldn't get out of bed. The therapist said, "First try to sit up; can you? "Yes," the patient replied. The therapist continued, "Now get out of bed. What's your usual morning routine?" The patient responded, "Well, I take a shower and have breakfast." The therapist went on, "So how about trying to stay with your usual daily routine; can you do it?"

In this example, the therapist not only gave advice but also encouraged the patient by structuring his behavior and reducing anxiety.

Therapist Self-Disclosure

The clinician should have a therapeutic rationale for any self-disclosure he or she engages in. Using personal experiences can provide opportunities for patients to identify with aspects of the therapist who may reveal certain attitudes and values. Such disclosure enables patients with ego deficits to build a more stable and cohesive sense of self and others. Straightforward answers to personal questions from the patient can be given within appropriate social conventions of privacy and reticence. Self-disclosure does have transference implications, but the therapist need not mention this to the patient. If a valid reason exists for self-disclosure, appropriate references to the therapist's experience and opinion may be helpful to the patient. In the following example, the therapist did not self-disclose, but instead behaved as if she were working in an expressive mode.

> A therapist in training was asked by a patient in supportive psychotherapy whether she liked to cook. The therapist sidestepped the question without responding. Her rationale was that answering the question would be too gratifying for the patient.

We believe that nonresponsiveness by the therapist in supportive psychotherapy, as illustrated in this example, can lead to heightened anxiety and unnecessary frustration for the patient. In contrast, self-disclosure is used less frequently in expressive psychotherapy, given that patients receiving this type of treatment generally possess a cohesive sense of self and other.

Cognitive-Behavioral Techniques

Cognitive-behavioral psychotherapy depends on clearly defined techniques designed to alter the way an individual thinks, appraises, and responds to events. The goals of cognitive-behavioral psychotherapy are to produce behavioral change and to reduce such symptoms as anxiety and depression by heightening the patient's awareness of negative thoughts or cognitive errors. Identifying and working on automatic thoughts helps to correct cognitive errors. Automatic thoughts are believed to originate from early learning experiences and from cognitive structures composed of relatively enduring beliefs and attitudes (termed *schemas*), which are challenged and restructured in treatment. Like supportive psychotherapy, cognitive-behavioral treatment focuses mainly on the present and emphasizes a collaborative and real relationship, rather than a transferential relationship.

Identifying and Examining Automatic Thoughts

Identifying and examining automatic thoughts are central techniques of cognitive therapy. Working on automatic thoughts leads to mastery and the development of structure. The therapeutic process involves identifying and challenging automatic beliefs and subjecting them to empirical testing. Patients are taught to monitor automatic thoughts, to question their validity, and to develop alternative ways of thinking. When patients learn that they can influence their thinking and change their cognitive responses, a sense of mastery is achieved. Automatic thoughts are habitual ways of experiencing and perceiving events and interpersonal interactions. These tend to be negative and often painful. Familiar examples of automatic thoughts include "If I am not married, then no one wants me" (or "I will never be happy"); "If I am not wealthy, then I am a failure"; "If my children are not successful, then I am an ineffectual parent"; "If I have an illness, then I did something wrong and deserve it."

> A patient who recently began working at a new location left his office building on a lunch-hour break but was afraid to explore his new surroundings. The therapist wondered aloud what the patient thought might happen if he ventured forth. "I might get lost and not be able to get back," the patient replied, and continued, "It doesn't make sense, I know it, but...that's how I feel." The automatic thought was identified and its validity was questioned. The patient was helped to understand the difference between his feeling and the fact of actually being lost (*decentering*).

Reframing

Reframing provides the patient with an alternative way of looking at an event that was previously perceived as painful or negative. It is useful in improving patient self-esteem, as illustrated below.

> A young mother complained that her toddler had started to run away from her and expressed her belief that the child was losing interest in her. A reframing of this painful and negative perception might be, "She feels secure enough with you so that she's free to explore the world."

Anticipatory Guidance

Anticipatory guidance is a useful technique for helping patients prepare for future encounters with situations perceived as potentially problematic. Preparation for a difficult event can be likened to studying for an examination or rehearsing for a performance. Gaining mastery over an anticipated situation diminishes anxiety and enhances self-efficacy.

An example of anticipatory guidance would be taking a patient through an initial telephone call to a prospective employer. The patient expects a cold reception and rejection. Rehearsal provides the patient with a number of scenarios and responses so that she will be equipped to cope with the anxiety engendered by making the telephone call and will have a repertoire of responses ready.

Relaxation and Breathing Techniques

Relaxation therapy is used to reduce anxiety. Explanation helps the patient understand that tension can exacerbate unpleasant situations and interfere with enjoyable activities. The patient is made aware of major muscle groups and how to tense and relax them. The technique of deep diaphragmatic breathing often is practiced in the session along with muscle relaxation. Patients should be instructed to perform this exercise twice a day and when symptoms of anxiety or panic occur to use deep breathing for a brief interval to ameliorate symptoms. Tension-producing situations need to be noted in a log book and discussed during therapy sessions.

Assertiveness Training

Assertiveness is the direct and positive expression of one's rights, thoughts, or feelings. Unexpressed thoughts or feelings tend to be indicative of passivity, while expressed thoughts or feelings can be assertive rather than aggressive if the feelings of others are considered. One important task is helping patients define assertion versus aggression and passivity. Four steps are used in promoting assertive behavior: 1) identify passive thoughts (e.g., "If I speak up, my boss won't like me"); 2) examine the positive and negative consequences of passive behavior; 3) work with patients on changing passive to assertive behavior and examine positive and negative consequences of assertive behavior; and 4) role playing (e.g., patient and therapist can role-play being direct and assertive with a supervisor).

Exposure Treatment

Exposure therapy is helpful for patients with pervasive anxiety and avoidance and is often used for the treatment of posttraumatic stress disorder (PTSD) and phobic problems. Exposure therapy can be in vivo or in vitro, depending on the nature of the problem. An in vivo approach can be used to desensitize patients to such things as phobias by direct exposure to the feared object or situation. An in vitro approach uses imaginal treatment (Foa 1997). The PTSD patient is asked to affectively relive and remember the traumatic event in great detail. The therapist empathically encourages, reassures, and educates the patient. Gradually, the trauma is detoxified, and the patient's memory of the event becomes organized as mistaken interpretations of the trauma are corrected. (An example of exposure therapy is presented in Case 2, "The Woman Who Thought She Was a Murderer" [Chapters 7, 8, and 9].)

Homework

Homework assignments function to extend the work of therapy beyond the session. Such assignments help patients to gather data and test hypotheses about themselves and the world so that dysfunctional thinking can be noted and modified. Examples of homework assignments include keeping a daily log of automatic thoughts, practicing techniques such as relaxation, reading a self-help book, joining a self-help group, and trying out new behaviors (e.g., making appointments with friends and/or meeting new people, being active rather than passive).

Patients' reactions to homework assignments should be elicited. How a patient reacts to an assignment will often add to the therapist's knowledge of the patient's underlying personality structure. For instance, a patient who fears criticism may not want to risk undertaking a homework assignment; for other patients, problems with homework may be based on misunderstanding the assignment and needing concrete help in undertaking the work.

Expressive Techniques

Like supportive treatment, expressive psychotherapy involves clearly defined techniques that have been developed to promote the exploration and affective and cognitive understanding of conflict, systems of belief, characteristic modes of responding and behaving, and personality problems. Although exploration is important in all psychotherapies, it forms the cornerstone of expressive psychotherapy techniques. Interventions are used to deepen and extend the exploratory process. Although patients may consciously want to behave in a different and more productive manner, they often unconsciously oppose the therapeutic process that will enable them to do so. Resistance and defensive behavior accompany the psychotherapy process every step of the way (Freud 1912/1958).

Exploration of resistance/defense is central to expressive psychotherapy. The two are linked, and in clinical settings they can be considered equivalent. The concept of resistance is specific to the therapy situation, whereas defense is ubiquitous and occurs both in and out of psychotherapy. Essentially, resistance in psychotherapy is expressed by defensive behavior. A number of techniques are useful in exploring resistance/defense.

Confrontation, Clarification, and Interpretation

These tools were defined earlier, in the section on supportive techniques. In expressive psychotherapy, confrontation, clarification, and interpretation are used somewhat differently than they are in supportive treatment. When resistance is encountered, it must be brought to the patient's attention. Confrontation is the technique used to make the patient aware of his or her resistance/defense.

The following vignettes illustrate the use of confrontation in expressive psychotherapy.

> A patient spoke of his girlfriend's having nursed him when he had the flu. His description was intellectualized and emotionless.
>
> > Therapist: She nursed you, but when you talk about her, it's without emotion or feeling.
>
> A patient was withdrawn and remote after his therapist returned from vacation. When the therapist asked the patient whether his behavior had anything to do with him (the therapist), the patient changed the subject.
>
> > Therapist: Do you notice that when I ask if your withdrawn behavior here has anything to do with me, you change the subject?

Clarification in expressive psychotherapy is used to explore resistance/defensive behavior after it has been brought to the patient's attention through the use of confrontation. In reality, confrontation and clarification are often used together. The therapist uses clarification to highlight the patient's elaboration of the therapist's confrontation.

In the second example above, the patient, after being confronted with his avoidance, went on to describe his thoughts about the therapist.

> Patient: I'm concerned about what you'll think of me if I complain about your vacation.

> Therapist: You're concerned about what I'll think of you if you complain, so you keep it to yourself and avoid your feelings toward me.

Interpretation provides an explanation for the patient's behavior. In brief expressive psychotherapy, interpretation is generally used in a broader fashion than in brief supportive psychotherapy. It can be directed at current and/or past relationships as well as at the therapeutic relationship. It is useful to think of the triangles of conflict and person when making interpretations in expressive psychotherapy (see Chapter 3). The following is an example of an interpretation with the patient described above.

> Patient: I worry about what you think of me. When you were away, I had a number of things I wanted to talk about, but I had no one to talk to. I was saying to myself, "Damn it, why does he have to be away now?"

> Therapist: So you were withdrawn and avoided talking about my vacation because you were irritated with me for being away when you had so much to talk about?

Cognitive-Behavioral and Dynamic Psychotherapy: Similarities and Differences

There are many similarities and differences between cognitive-behavioral and dynamic treatments of the expressive and supportive types, and these need to be understood by therapists who use an integrated approach. Understanding these differences and similarities will help therapists think more clearly about differential therapeutics so that the most appropriate and efficacious techniques are used regardless of their therapy derivation. In addition, it will help guide the clinician when transitioning between therapies, which will be discussed at the end of this chapter.

A number of major points of congruence exist among therapeutic approaches. Six common elements have been described (A. Winston and Muran 1996): 1) expression of feelings and thoughts (Rosenzweig 1936); 2) self-examination and self-understanding (Rosenzweig 1936); 3) provision of a rationale that includes a plausible system of explanation of the patient's problems or distress (Frank and Frank 1991); 4) strengthening the patient's expectations of help—the arousal of hope (Frank and Frank 1991); 5) encouragement of mastery efforts and testing of different approaches and solutions (Lambert 1986); and 6) the patient-therapist or helping relationship (Frank and Frank 1991).

The expression of feelings and thoughts is connected to the concept of the corrective emotional experience (Alexander and French 1946). Originally applied to dynamic psychotherapy, this concept refers to the opportunity therapy affords the patient to reexperience an aspect of a difficult problem or conflictual relationship from the past with a benign figure in the present—the therapist. Alexander (1963) later applied aspects of learning theory to this concept, expanding its scope to include any confrontation with a problematic issue from which a patient could learn to master or cope with that issue. In cognitive-behavioral therapy, the use of exposure techniques provides a corrective experience.

Self-examination and self-understanding are applied in most forms of psychotherapy and aid in developing a rationale for the patient's problems. Providing a plausible explanatory system is an important part of many therapies. For example, dynamic psychotherapy searches for underlying wishes that may not be conscious to explain certain types of behavior, whereas cognitive treatment seeks out underlying beliefs or schema to understand current thinking.

The expectation or hope that psychotherapy will prove helpful when other efforts have failed can lead to more successful treatment (Frank and Frank 1991). Many patients enter psychotherapy in a demoralized state, but this can change when they are offered hope (Shapiro 1981). Without a doubt, hope is an important element in both cognitive-behavioral and dynamic therapies.

Changing maladaptive behavior and thinking by helping patients face fears and difficult problems, explore different solutions to these problems, and execute strategies to solve problems all help promote mastery, or cognitive control. Cognitive therapy attempts to promote mastery by designing graduated tasks with well-defined goals so that the patient can experience success (Beck et al. 1979). Psychodynamic therapies attempt to promote adaptation and mastery by improving ego function and by utilization of the working-through process. The working-through process involves repeated exploration of an insight into new situations and with different people. Bandura (1982) discussed mastery in terms of *self-efficacy,* which refers to the belief that one can successfully execute a given behavior.

The sixth common factor, the patient-therapist relationship, may be the most important (Hartley 1985; Horvath and Symonds 1991; A. Winston and Muran 1996). Dynamic therapy consistently emphasizes the importance of the therapeutic relationship and in its expressive form uses transference interpretations to facilitate the exploratory process (see Chapter 4). Although also dynamic, supportive therapy addresses the patient-therapist relationship only when it becomes problematic. In the past, cognitive-behavioral therapists treated the therapeutic relationship as a background condition, to be explored only if it interfered with treatment. In recent years, however, there has been a greater interest in and use of the therapeutic relationship, particularly by "master" cognitive-behavioral therapists (Goldfried et al. 1998).

Many factors distinguish cognitive-behavioral from dynamic expressive therapy (Blagys and Hilsenroth 2000). Supportive therapy, although dynamically based, is closer to cognitive-behavioral therapy in its practice. Emotion and affect are emphasized in expressive therapy, whereas cognitive-behavioral and supportive treatments focus more on thoughts than on feelings. In expressive treatment, attention to the past and how it influences present difficulties is an integral part of the therapy. In cognitive-behavioral and supportive therapies, the primary focus is the patient's present life. That being said, it is also true that cognitive-behavioral therapists have recently become more interested in exploring the origins of dysfunctional thinking (Young 1999).

Cognitive-behavioral therapists have not traditionally focused on hindrances to the progress of therapy. Expressive therapy explores patient resistance to uncover its meaning and impact on the therapeutic relationship. In supportive treatment, the therapist may address avoidance only in extreme circumstances, such as when the patient-therapist relationship or the therapy is threatened. At other times, the patient may avoid painful material, which the therapist generally will not address because it may be too threatening to the patient.

Whereas cognitive-behavioral and supportive therapies emphasize symptom reduction, expressive therapy with an interpersonal focus is concerned with maladaptive patterns of interpersonal relationships and issues of the self. Cognitive-behavioral therapy advocates use of homework to promote change and further the work of therapy between sessions. It also stresses strengthening of the patient's coping ability to promote present and future functioning when problematic events and experiences are encountered.

A final distinguishing element of expressive therapy is the exploration of dreams, fantasies, and wishes. Supportive and cognitive-behavioral therapies typically do not explore these issues.

Transitioning Between Approaches

Transitioning between expressive, supportive, and cognitive-behavioral therapies requires an understanding of these approaches, their similarities and differences, and the patient's position on the psychological structure/psychotherapy continuum. As the therapist shifts back and forth between approaches, explanations need to be given to the patient to facilitate the transition process. Transitioning is also very important when a combined approach of psychotherapy and pharmacotherapy is used.

Many supportive techniques are used in expressive psychotherapy. However, with higher-functioning patients, techniques such as giving advice, praise, and encouragement are rarely employed. As noted earlier, we find that most patients lie near the midpoint of the continuum and require a blend of supportive and expressive approaches. A major challenge for the therapist is to determine whether to use a supportive or an expressive approach in a given situation with a given patient. Wallace (1983) captured the essence of this dilemma:

> It is difficult to decide which response is correct. You cannot wait for the patient to make connections....You must decide...now to come down on the side of expressiveness, now of restraint, now to confront his intellectualization or reaction formation, now to support it, now to analyze the transference, now to utilize it as a suggestive or reinforcing lever...now to ask him what goes into his question, now to answer it immediately and directly, now to gratify his request for coffee or advice, now to analyze it. (pp. 345–346)

Some of the challenges of transitioning are illustrated in the following vignette:

> A patient at the midpoint of the psychological structure/psychotherapy continuum has been exploring her relationships with significant people in her life. She began a session by reporting the sudden death of her sister-in-law. There was an exploration of the patient's feelings about her sister-in-law and the impact of her death on the patient's husband and children. Later in the session, the patient asked the therapist whether she should bring her children, ages 12 and 14, to the funeral. This question represented a decision point for the therapist. Should there be a direct answer,

some exploration of this question and no direct answer, or exploration followed by advice? The therapist responded, "I'll tell you what I think, but let's take a few minutes to understand your thoughts and feelings about it."

Often, after exploration of an issue of this type, patients are able to reach a conclusion themselves. At other times, patients will require an answer from the therapist:

The patient, after some exploration, was unable to make a decision until the therapist said, "Most children who willingly accompany their families to a funeral of a family member do not have adverse reactions; in fact, going to a funeral and burial can provide closure and enable children to mourn with their families."

Transitioning can also involve a shift from supportive therapy to expressive treatment, as in the example below:

Another patient entered treatment with a severe major depressive disorder, following several losses, including her job and boyfriend. Antidepressant medication and brief supportive psychotherapy were started. The therapist encouraged the patient to be more active, to follow a regular routine, and to make social engagements. Cognitive measures, including identification and examination of automatic thoughts, were undertaken. By the sixth week the patient was improved but stated that she wanted to understand why she repeatedly had problems with men and at work. A shift to a more expressive approach was initiated by the therapist. The therapist said: "Now that your depression is better, it would be helpful if we can explore your thoughts, difficulties, feelings, and relationships, so that we can understand the conflicts and maladaptive patterns in your life and help you to do something about them."

Conclusions

We have discussed a number of techniques used in supportive, cognitive-behavioral, and expressive forms of brief psychotherapy. Because the full application of these and other techniques cannot be readily encapsulated in brief clinical vignettes, the reader is referred to Chapters 7, 8, and 9, in which comprehensive discussions and additional examples of technical interventions are provided.

CHAPTER

6

The Partnership
Medication and Psychotherapy

The title of this chapter constitutes a recognition that the beginning of a real partnership is now possible between psychotherapy and pharmacotherapy. Attitudes of the public and mental health professionals have ranged between attempts to build bridges between the opposing parties and overt hostility. At the same time, practicing psychiatrists, social workers, psychologists, and nurses have participated in combined treatments for many years. Most clinicians recognize that many patients require both drug treatment and psychotherapy (M. Sullivan et al. 1993). If this is the case, why has there been so much difficulty with combined treatment?

The answer appears to lie in the attitudes and ideologies of both professionals and patients. Some psychiatrists with a biological orientation disparage psychotherapy; other psychiatrists and not a few nonmedical therapists view medication with skepticism or feel that its use may interfere with psychotherapy. Some patients enter treatment believing that they have a "chemical imbalance" and ask for medication; others refuse medication that would greatly relieve their suffering on the grounds that its use would constitute a weakness.

In the past, a number of interactions between drug treatment and psychotherapy, some positive and some negative, were hypothesized (Klerman

1991). On the negative side, it was believed that adding drug treatment to psychotherapy would interfere with the therapeutic relationship or decrease motivation for psychotherapy when symptoms disappeared. However, Weissman (1979), reviewing studies in which depressed patients were treated with psychotherapy alone, pharmacotherapy alone, and psychotherapy in combination with pharmacotherapy, found no negative interactions. Rounsaville et al. (1981), in a clinical trial of psychotherapy and a tricyclic antidepressant (TCA), also found no evidence to support hypotheses predicting negative interactions with combined treatments.

On the positive side, medication may enable patients to be more receptive to psychotherapy, and psychotherapy may increase patients' receptivity to medication. For example, patients with severe mood disorders are generally unable to engage in psychotherapy because their conscious awareness is impaired. With improved mood, receptivity to and interaction with the therapist and with the therapeutic interventions are more likely. A number of studies support the efficacy of a combined approach. For instance, combination treatment can improve medication compliance (Goodwin and Jamison 1990), decrease relapse (Hogarty et al. 1997), and reduce readmission rates (Clarkin et al. 1990). In addition, Vaughan and colleagues (1997) found that medication can increase motivation and psychological mindedness. They also reported that patients with Axis I disorders drop out of treatment less often when receiving combined treatment than when receiving psychotherapy alone.

Efficacy Studies

The evidence for the efficacy of psychopharmacological treatments in psychiatric conditions such as major depressive disorder, panic disorder, bipolar disorder, and schizophrenia is well established. Innumerable clinical trials have demonstrated the usefulness of drugs in these disorders. The evidence for the efficacy of psychotherapy for a number of psychiatric disorders, including major depressive disorder, panic disorder, obsessive-compulsive disorder, posttraumatic stress disorder, and personality disorders, has become more convincing in recent years (see Chapter 10 for a discussion of psychotherapy research).

Integrated or combined approaches have not been studied extensively for most disorders, with the possible exception of major depressive disorder. We conducted a review of the research literature published since 1976 on combined treatment. In the following sections we summarize some of the major studies and reviews, as well as clinical reports and proposed approaches.

Major Depressive Disorder

Weissman (1979) identified 17 clinical trials conducted in homogeneous samples of depressed outpatients that examined the efficacy of psychotherapy alone, psychotherapy versus pharmacotherapy, and—in 4 of these studies—psychotherapy in combination with pharmacotherapy. In the 4 studies of combined treatment, which involved moderately ill depressed patients, the effects of therapy and medication were found to be additive; no negative interactions were reported. Blackburn et al. (1981), examining a sample of nonbipolar depressed patients drawn from an outpatient tertiary care setting, found that drug treatment combined with cognitive therapy was superior to either single modality. In the same study but a different sample (patients from a general practice setting), these investigators found that cognitive therapy, either alone or in combination with drug therapy, was superior to pharmacotherapy alone. However, there was some indication that drug treatment provided by the general practitioners was less than optimal. Conte et al. (1986) examined 17 published reports on 11 controlled studies of combined therapy for major depressive disorder. They concluded that combined treatment was superior to either psychotherapy or drug treatment alone but that the effect was not a strong one. Reynolds et al. (1992), using nortriptyline and interpersonal psychotherapy for approximately 25 weeks of acute and continuation therapy, reported a good response and a relatively low attrition rate in elderly patients with recurrent major depression. In a later controlled clinical trial lasting 16 weeks, Reynolds and colleagues (1999) found that the combination of nortriptyline and interpersonal therapy (versus nortriptyline alone, interpersonal therapy alone, or placebo) was associated with the highest rate of treatment completion in patients with bereavement-related major depressive episodes.

The studies described above all indicate an advantage for combined treatment in comparison with either psychotherapy or medication alone. However, other studies (Jarrett 1995; Shea et al. 1988) have suggested that the combination of medication and psychotherapy is not superior to either modality alone, and the Depression Guideline Panel (1993) reported that combination treatments are roughly equal to pharmacotherapy alone for acute-phase treatment. In their review, Shea and colleagues added the caveat that because the sample sizes were small and single modalities were quite effective, there was little room for combined treatment to show a significant advantage. In addition, they described other studies (discussed below) that appear to demonstrate an advantage for combined treatment when a broader domain of outcome (e.g., social adjustment) is considered. Jarrett (1995), in his discussion, also listed some reservations, stating that if patients prefer combination treatment to either treatment alone, combined treatment may be more effective when efficacy measures include dropout rates, compliance, and intention-to-treat analysis (patients who dropped out were included in the overall outcome analysis).

Investigators have examined a number of additional factors regarding outcome with combined versus single treatments. Two studies found that combined treatment with behavioral therapy and medication produced improvement significantly more rapidly than did behavioral treatment alone (Roth et al. 1982; Wilson 1982). In addition, combined treatment may have a broader effect, working on both symptoms and social adjustment (A. S. Friedman 1975; Weissman 1979; Weissman et al. 1976, 1981).

Sotsky et al. (1991) reported that specific patient characteristics, such as social, cognitive, and work function, may predict which patients with major depressive disorder will respond best to which treatments. In their study, for example, low social dysfunction predicted superior response to interpersonal therapy (IPT); low cognitive dysfunction predicted superior response to cognitive-behavioral therapy (CBT); and high work dysfunction, high depression severity, and impairment of function predicted superior response to imipramine and to IPT. Although Sotsky and colleagues did not examine combined treatments, their findings suggest the possibility of tailoring treatment approaches to patient characteristics in addition to diagnosis.

Using a "mega-analysis" method, Thase et al. (1997) found that combined therapy (IPT or CBT plus medication) was superior to psychotherapy alone for the treatment of severe, recurrent depression. Combined therapy was not significantly more effective than psychotherapy alone in milder depressions, however. In another article, Thase (1997) concluded that combined therapy is not routinely indicated for uncomplicated major depression and provided examples of circumstances in which combined therapy can have a profound effect.

In the largest investigation of combined treatments to date, Keller et al. (2000) studied 681 patients with chronic depression treated for 12 weeks with nefazodone (antidepressant) alone, a cognitive-behavioral analysis system of psychotherapy (CBASP) alone, or combined nefazodone and CBASP. The response rates for the first 12 weeks (acute phase) of treatment were 55% for nefazodone alone, 52% for CBASP alone, and 85% for the combined therapy.

The studies reviewed here appear to indicate that a combined approach is most advantageous for severe, recurrent depression or chronic depression and perhaps also for depression in the elderly. For acute and nonrecurrent depression, however, combination treatment may not have an advantage—except perhaps through its possible broader effect, particularly on social adjustment. In the studies cited above, the lack of findings supporting superior effects for combined treatment may in part be the result of the studies' failure to separate patients with depressive disorder according to illness severity or chronicity, or of the studies' exclusive focus on symptom reduction, an aspect of outcome that may not be enhanced with combined treatment.

Other Psychiatric Disorders

Combined approaches in schizophrenia have produced some positive results. Psychodynamic therapy has generally been ineffective for individuals with this illness, for a number of reasons. Case management with an assertive community approach helps retain patients in treatment programs and keep them out of the hospital, but its effect on functioning is unremarkable (Bond et al. 1995). Social skills training can delay relapse and improve adjustment (Benton and Schroeder 1990). Gunderson et al. (1984) reported that supportive therapy produced a decrease in recidivism as compared with a more expressive psychotherapy. Hogarty and colleagues (1997) conducted a 3-year trial of "personal therapy" in 151 patients with schizophrenia or schizoaffective disorder who were receiving antipsychotic medication. This therapy model involves the use of a graduated three-stage systemic approach to identify affective, cognitive, and physiological experiences of stress. Hogarty et al. reported that for patients living with family, but not those living independently, personal therapy was effective in preventing psychotic and affective relapse as well as noncompliance. Sensky and colleagues (2000) reported that CBT resulted in significant improvement in schizophrenic patients who were resistant to antipsychotics. Both positive and negative symptoms diminished during the 9-month follow-up.

In a review of psychotherapy for bipolar disorder, Jamison (1991) concluded that psychotherapy can be of unique value to patients undergoing the devastating changes of the illness. As with schizophrenia, combining medication with psychotherapy can result in better drug compliance and more favorable clinical outcomes (Cochran 1984; Glick et al. 1985). Post (1992) suggested that different psychosocial and psychotherapeutic interventions, together with pharmacotherapy, might be used, depending on the stage of the illness. In particular, early intervention may help prevent rapid cycling, spontaneous episodes, and refractoriness to drug treatment. For example, psychodynamic therapy may be appropriate for early, "minor stress-related dysphorias or initial episodes of major depression" (Post 1992, p. 1006), whereas cognitive, interpersonal, and behavioral therapies may be better when repeated episodes emerge. Miklowitz (1996) reported results from a family-focused psychoeducational treatment and an individual, interpersonally oriented psychotherapy that suggest high retention rates over the first year of treatment for both approaches.

Hohagen et al. (1998), studying patients with obsessive-compulsive disorder, reported that multimodal behavior therapy combined with fluvoxamine (a selective serotonin reuptake inhibitor [SSRI] antidepressant) was significantly superior to multimodal behavior therapy plus placebo in patients with severe obsessions or secondary severe depression. For compulsions, there were no significant differences between the two treatment conditions.

In a study of bulimia nervosa, Walsh et al. (1997) reported that whereas CBT is the psychological treatment of choice for this condition, fluoxetine (an SSRI) adds modestly to the benefit of CBT. Compared with CBT alone, the combined approach produced greater improvement in binge eating and depression.

In posttraumatic stress disorder, the expert consensus guidelines point to psychotherapy as the treatment of choice for mild to moderately impaired patients (Foa et al. 1999). Suggested techniques include exposure, anxiety management, and cognitive treatment. For patients with more severe symptoms, the experts were divided. Whereas the medical experts preferred combination therapy, the psychotherapy experts felt that psychotherapy alone was the best choice.

Carroll and colleagues (1995), in a study of depressed versus nondepressed cocaine abusers treated with desipramine (an antidepressant of the tricyclic type) and CBT, found that desipramine was effective in reducing depressive symptoms but not cocaine use. CBT produced more consecutive days of abstinence and better treatment retention in the depressed group but did not have an effect on depressive symptoms. Carroll et al. concluded that the two treatments produced differential symptom reduction in depressed cocaine addicts, a finding that underscores the importance of evaluating combined treatments. In a later article, Carroll (1997) suggested that "for many substance use disorders, outcomes can be broadened, enhanced and extended by combining the most effective forms of psychotherapy and pharmacotherapy" (p. 233).

Medically Ill Patients

In a review of studies spanning 30 years, Twillman and Manetto (1998) concluded that a combined approach was somewhat more effective than monotherapy in treating various psychiatric disorders and preventing relapse. They reviewed treatment approaches for depression and outlined reasons why a combined approach might be the preferred model for intervening with depressed cancer patients. Muskin (1990) also called attention to the combined use of psychotherapy and pharmacotherapy in the medical setting. He suggested that psychiatrists who consult in medical settings must attend to both psychodynamic and psychopharmacological issues.

In summary, combined treatment may have an advantage over medication alone or psychotherapy alone in reducing symptoms in some disorders. In addition, a combined approach may have broader effects, benefiting interpersonal relations and social adjustment and improving medication compliance. There is now some evidence indicating that drug treatment in combination with psychotherapy leads to symptom reduction in chronic depression and severe recurrent depression, but not in mild or moderate major depression.

Much more research is needed on combined treatment for most psychiatric disorders. It is important to realize that efficacy studies are based on clinical trials, which are designed to treat homogeneous groups of patients. Therefore, patients with comorbid disorders and other complicating conditions may be excluded from these studies. Today, comorbidity is more likely the rule than the exception (Kessler et al. 1994; Regier et al. 1990). A multimodal treatment approach incorporating psychotherapy and medication may be needed with this population. "Real world" problems need to be taken into account by designing studies that are less rarefied and exclusionary. Recent efforts in this regard in the form of services or effectiveness research that studies "real world" problems may address these deficiencies. In the meantime, in the absence of more definitive studies of combined treatment for each psychiatric disorder, clinicians must rely on clinical judgment to select the appropriate treatment approach.

Psychopharmacology-Psychotherapy Integration

As therapists begin the process of treatment planning, the option of combined treatment generally should be considered. A unified approach to treatment offers a greater range of options. Not all patients need medication, but many will benefit from it. The decision to use medication should be based on a thorough evaluation of the patient and the latest findings from clinical trials and real-life studies. Whether medication will be recommended depends on a number of considerations, such as diagnosis, severity of illness, and the behavioral dimensions exhibited by the patient. Examples of behavioral dimensions include agitation, impulsivity, psychosis, and mood. Regardless of the diagnosis, behavioral dimensions and their severities must be considered and may be more important than diagnosis. For example, a patient with a major depressive disorder of mild severity may need only psychotherapy, whereas a patient with severe recurrent or chronic depression will probably require a combined approach (Keller et al. 2000; Thase et al. 1997). A patient with a psychotic depression most likely will need psychotherapy and both an antipsychotic for the behavioral dimension of psychosis and an antidepressant to treat the severe disorder of mood (Charney and Nelson 1981; Nelson and Bowers 1978).

How a clinician perceives the integration of pharmacotherapy and psychotherapy will influence the overall therapeutic process. Therapists may have positive or negative thoughts, attitudes, and feelings regarding the use of medication, as well as countertransference issues. Some therapists will view the introduction of medication into a psychotherapy as a defeat; other therapists will perceive medication as a crutch. Beitman (1981) cautioned against envisioning a strict dichotomy between verbal and drug approaches. He suggested that pharmacotherapy should instead be thought of as only one of many interventions available to the therapist, stating that "[m]edications, like verbal interventions, may help or hinder engagement, resistance, transference, countertransference and working through" (Beitman 1981, p. 206).

Goldhammer (1983) called attention to the "interactive effects" of combined therapy as essential in alleviating symptoms and enriching interpersonal experience. He emphasized the importance of patients' interpersonal concerns related to medication use. These concerns can be played out within the patient-therapist relationship and may involve rejection, manipulation, acceptance, or narcissistic injury.

Therefore, when pharmacotherapy is introduced, changed, or terminated, the patient-therapist relationship may be affected. The clinician, as always, must monitor the therapeutic relationship so that a positive alliance is maintained (see Chapter 4). When problems such as rejection of medication, missed appointments, noncompliance, feelings of being misunderstood, or any other indicators of an alliance breach occur, the clinician should address these issues in the patient-therapist relationship and explore their connection with the medication.

> Maria, a 27-year-old woman with a diagnosis of borderline personality disorder, had been in psychotherapy for 6 weeks. Her parasuicidal behavior of cutting her forearms began to increase and a number of depressive symptoms emerged. At this point, her therapist suggested a consultation with a

psychiatrist to evaluate her need for medication. After missing the next psychotherapy session the patient was asked how she felt about being sent for a medication consultation. The patient reported that she thought the therapist was giving up on her by suggesting a medication evaluation.

Although breaks in the alliance are not uncommon in the treatment of patients with severe personality disorder, this break might have been avoided if the therapist had immediately engaged the patient in an exploration of her thoughts and feelings about the consultation and its meaning.

There are no controlled studies of combined treatment of patients with borderline personality disorder; however, Koenigsberg (1991) pointed out that medication can be useful for treating some of the common behavioral dimensions in this population. We have found that borderline personality disorder patients with mood instability and irritability can become more accessible to psychotherapy when treated with SSRIs.

Sequencing

A combined approach can either be used from the beginning of treatment or be implemented at some point during treatment. The addition of psychotherapy to an ongoing pharmacotherapeutic treatment has been called *sequencing*.

A number of factors should be considered in the decision to use a sequencing approach. First, mood can significantly affect cognition and perception. How one experiences oneself, others, the future, and the environment is thought to be related to mood.

Ted, a 49-year-old man with severe major depression, had significant cognitive impairment. He was unable to engage in a give-and-take relationship and could respond only to simple questions. After several weeks on an antidepressant, he became more responsive and was able to engage in psychotherapy in a productive manner.

Second, once symptoms are ameliorated with medication, character structure and personality issues can be more readily discerned.

Ted initially appeared passive, needy, and dependent. When his depression lifted, however, it became clear that he was not a passive, dependent man, but rather an assertive individual who could be quite independent.

This change in Ted is in keeping with the clinical adage that a personality diagnosis (Axis II) should not be made in the presence of significant Axis I psychopathology.

Third, symptoms can be debilitating and can affect self-esteem, leading to pessimism. When symptoms diminish, self-esteem often improves, and the individual becomes more optimistic. This change can increase motivation for and receptivity to psychotherapy.

Finally, it should be noted that the patient-therapist relationship is different in pharmacotherapy than in psychotherapy. Less responsibility is assigned to patients in pharmacotherapy, while patients in psychotherapy are expected to work as actively as possible.

Integrated Versus Split Treatment

Integrated treatment is defined as psychotherapy and pharmacotherapy provided by a psychiatrist. *Split treatment* refers to pharmacotherapy supplied by a psychiatrist and psychotherapy provided by a nonphysician therapist. A survey in the Seattle area found that 63% of psychiatrists participate in split treatment with nonphysicians (Beitman et al. 1984). Unfortunately, this arrangement reinforces a mind/brain duality, with the psychiatrist concentrating on the brain and the social worker or psychologist on the mind. In the best practice approach, synthesis of mind/brain can be achieved with a psychiatrist providing both treatments or a highly collaborative relationship between the nonmedical therapist and psychiatrist.

Two reasons have been suggested for the growing prevalence of collaborative treatment. The first is the "medicalization" of psychiatry, in that psychiatrists are increasingly being required to concentrate on pharmacotherapy at the expense of psychotherapy. The second is the emergence of managed care, with its emphasis on cost reduction. Two studies have compared the costs of integrated and split treatments. In the first study (Goldman et al. 1998), patients receiving integrated treatment received significantly fewer sessions and had lower treatment costs on average than did those in split treatment. The second study (Dewan 1999) used the fee schedules of 7 large managed care organizations to model expenses for psychotherapy alone, medication alone, and either an integrated treatment provided by a psychiatrist or a split treatment provided by a psychiatrist and a psychologist or social worker. Brief psychotherapy conducted by a social worker was the least expensive. Integrated treatment provided by a psychiatrist cost about the same or was less expensive than split treatment with a social worker and was usually less expensive than split treatment with a psychologist. These two studies seem to indicate that cost should not be a major consideration when weighing the merits of integrated versus collaborative approaches.

In an effort to reframe the "split," we will refer to treatment by two professionals as "collaborative" treatment. A successful collaborative relationship should be open, with easy access for communication so that both therapists and the patient are working on agreed-upon treatment goals. The monitoring of medication compliance and side effects is an important component of pharmacotherapy. In a collaborative relationship, both therapists need to be mindful of these issues. Because medication noncompliance and side effects can potentially undermine treatment, attending to these areas is just as important for the nonmedical therapist as it is for the pharmacotherapist.

The following is an example of medication noncompliance.

> Martin, a 42-year-old man with major depressive disorder and a number of interpersonal problems, was in a collaborative treatment. After 5 weeks on an antidepressant medication, his depression lifted and Martin and his therapist began to explore interpersonal problems. In the seventh week, the therapist noticed that Martin was having difficulty concentrating and appeared less energetic. It became clear that his depression was returning, so the therapist asked about Martin's use of the antidepressant. Martin revealed that he had stopped the medication because he thought he was over his depression. Although education on medication use had been provided earlier in treatment, Martin's sense of well-being overrode past educative efforts. At this point, the therapist initiated an exploration of Martin's motivations in discontinuing his medication. What emerged were the patient's concerns about needing to "rely" on something artificial and outside himself, which he thought made him weak and less of a man.

Side effects of medication can lead to noncompliance and can have a negative effect on the patient-therapist relationship, as illustrated below.

> Barbara, a 32-year-old woman with a highly refractory form of obsessive-compulsive disorder, experienced a dramatic improvement of her symptoms on a regimen of sertraline (an SSRI), clomipramine (a TCA), and cognitive-behavioral treatment. However, she began to complain to her nonmedical therapist that she no longer derived pleasure from having sexual relations with her husband. Although she had been told that the medication might have sexual side effects, Barbara was concerned that something was wrong with her physically. The therapist reassured Barbara by explaining that her symptoms were a medication side effect and consulted with the pharmacotherapist to address the problem.

Collaborative relationships between medical and nonmedical therapists can work in the best interests of the patient. However, it should be kept in mind that these relationships can become conflictual. A major problem is inadequate communication. There are several contact points that are crucial for a successful collaboration. When the initial referral is made, active, direct communication should take place between the nonmedical and the medical therapist. Other necessary contact points are after the initial evaluation, after changes in medication and dosage, in the event of significant side effects, and in the event of medication noncompliance. Collaboration is especially important during the termination process, because questions about long-term medication maintenance or discontinuation of medication need to be discussed at that time.

Other conflictual problems may occur between the medical and the non-medical therapist. These include competition, jealousy, and splitting. In this sense, a triangular relationship exists among the three participants (Carli 1999). Both therapists need to understand the nature of triangular relationships and the potential for conflict.

> Gail, a 41-year-old woman, complained to her therapist that her pharma-cotherapist was big, scary, and tough. She asked to be referred to another pharmacotherapist. After consulting with the second pharmacotherapist, however, she reported feeling misunderstood and ignored, in contrast to her feelings about her psychotherapist, whom she liked and tended to ide-alize. Exploration of Gail's conflict revealed a need for an exclusive rela-tionship with her therapist. The pharmacotherapist represented a threat to this dyadic relationship.

In a triangular conflict, communication between the therapists as well as exploration of the patient's conflict will clarify the underlying dynamic constellation and provide the patient with a therapeutic experience.

Conclusions

At present, a combination of psychotherapy and pharmacotherapy may be the treatment of choice for a number of psychiatric disorders. Severity of ill-ness and behavioral dimensions such as mood or psychosis may be more im-portant than diagnosis in determining the need for combined treatment. While there are some advantages to having one therapist provide both treat-ments, collaborative treatment approaches with a pharmacotherapist and psychotherapist are often the rule. That being the case, the relationship be-tween the two therapists should be one of open and respectful communica-tion, with a number of contact points, as outlined above.

7

Initial Phase of Treatment

Treatment begins when therapist and patient meet. The therapist promotes rapport by providing a therapeutic experience that begins with the evaluation or first session. Ideally, a therapeutic process is initiated that can ultimately enable the patient to achieve his or her goals. It goes without saying that the therapist needs to be knowledgeable, understanding, empathic, and genuine. He or she must convey a positive regard for the patient.

The therapist's office should be thoughtfully planned, comfortable, and inviting. In the first session, the fee should be discussed, including methods of billing and payment. In addition, insurance matters such as release of information forms, managed care issues, confidentiality, and length of treatment need to be addressed. In brief integrated treatment, sessions are 45 to 50 minutes in length and generally are held weekly.

As goals are formulated, an explanation of the treatment process is in order. This includes the roles of the patient and therapist, scheduling, vacations, and missed sessions. Therapist flexibility with regard to vacations and missed sessions is essential. For patients on the left side of the psychopathology–psychological structure continuum (i.e., those with more psychopathology), attempts should be made to reschedule missed appointments. If the therapist rigidly holds to a payment requirement for missed sessions, patients who have not achieved object constancy may be unable to maintain a positive therapeutic relationship and may prematurely terminate treatment (Blanck and Blanck 1974). Patients on the right side of the continuum (i.e., those with more structure) may miss a session for a variety of reasons. Again, the therapist should be flexible and attempt to reschedule. At times, sessions will be missed for frivolous reasons. In these instances, patients generally should be held to the payment arrangement.

In the initial session, the therapist explains what the patient can expect from the therapist and what the patient's role will be.

> Charles, a 30-year-old man, sought therapy because of significant relationship problems with women. At the end of the evaluation, the therapist outlined what the patient could expect from treatment: "I'm going to try to help you understand yourself, your problems, your thinking processes, and what gets in your way. We agreed that one of your goals is to develop a close relationship with a woman. As we saw today, your problems with your mother and father are related to this difficulty." The therapist must speak naturally and avoid intellectualization when spelling out the patient's role in therapy: "If you can speak as openly as possible about your thoughts and feelings, yourself, and your relationships, then we can work together to help you make the changes that will enable you to achieve your goals."

As part of setting the stage for a positive therapeutic relationship, the patient is invited to discuss thoughts and feelings about the therapist or the therapy during the course of treatment. Therapists should be aware that most patients find it difficult to talk about their feelings and thoughts toward the therapist, even when encouraged to do so (see Chapter 4).

A thorough assessment of the patient's psychological functioning and response to trial therapy will establish the individual's position on the psychological structure/psychotherapy continuum. This process generally should be completed within the first two sessions of psychotherapy. The patient's major problems are identified, and therapy begins. The therapist's technical approach will be based on this assessment.

In this chapter and the two chapters that follow it, we use the cases of four patients at different points on the psychological structure/psychotherapy continuum to illustrate supportive, expressive, and combined approaches. The assessment and the initial phase of therapy are covered in the remainder of this chapter. The midphase and termination phase of treatment will be described in Chapters 8 and 9, respectively. It should be understood that "pure" forms of expressive or supportive psychotherapy do not exist.

Supportive elements are present in expressive therapy, and some exploration occurs in therapy that is highly supportive. For patients on both sides of the continuum, cognitive-behavioral techniques should be used to address problems such as dysfunctional thinking, severe anxiety, and irrational fears. Many cognitive-behavioral approaches are highly didactic and include explication of the therapeutic model and the rationale for interventions that are undertaken. Integration of these approaches (supportive, expressive, and cognitive-behavioral) should become seamless as the clinician becomes increasingly comfortable using the various interventions outlined in Chapter 5.

As each case unfolds, the therapist should pay particular attention to the therapeutic relationship as an essential ingredient of psychotherapy. As discussed in Chapter 4, the therapeutic relationship includes the therapeutic alliance and both transference and countertransference issues.

During the initial phase of psychotherapy, following the assessment, the therapist continues to learn about the patient's life. For patients on the supportive side of the psychotherapy continuum, the emphasis is on current life, as opposed to the past. Attention is given to decreasing anxiety and arousal so that the patient can work in psychotherapy. Many patients on the supportive side of the continuum will benefit from medication. Individuals with Axis I diagnoses such as major depression or panic disorder or severe Axis II diagnoses may require medication. For patients on the expressive side of the psychotherapy continuum, the emphasis is on relational issues and uncovering the basis and source of conflict. Increased arousal and anxiety is not avoided and can be helpful in furthering the uncovering process by causing enough discomfort in the patient to foster change. The heightening of anxiety and arousal creates a "temporary disorganization...and subsequent restructuring within a functional frame" (Hoehn-Saric 1978, p. 104). As patients in supportive psychotherapy change and improve, therapy may become more expressive. At times a more supportive approach may be required when a patient cannot tolerate interpretative work. Adjusting the treatment approach to the needs of the patient requires flexibility.

Case 1: Supportive Psychotherapy— The Woman Who Lived on the Edge

Lucy, a 34-year-old African-American married woman, was referred for treatment 8 weeks after the birth of her second daughter. She identified her major problem as a sense that her life was falling apart and having a dead and empty feeling inside. She was suicidal and sleep deprived and had lost 15 pounds.

A friend brought her for the initial visit because she was unable to come alone. Although anxious and uneasy at first, Lucy was open and honest with the therapist about her life. She has been married for 12 years, has an 11-year-old daughter Brenda, and has been having an affair for the past 3 years. Lucy has mixed feelings toward her lover, John, who at times seems attentive to her, but who also is abusive, rejecting, and inconsistent.

She described her husband, Carl, as a good man who cared enormously about his older daughter. She had married him because he was educated, intelligent, and hardworking. However, from the beginning of their marriage, he had spent a great deal of time away from home, either at work or with his friends. Lucy had difficulty managing when her husband was away from home. At night she often walked the streets looking for him, leaving her daughter Brenda, then an infant, home alone.

From infancy on, Lucy's life had been replete with losses and changes in caretakers. As a child, she had been physically and sexually abused. After spending the first 3 years of life with her grandparents, Lucy was returned to her mother. At age 5, she was sent to her father, who was a kind man but away from home for long periods of time. During his absences, Lucy was mistreated by his callous and brutal wife.

Session 1

The patient came to the first session with a friend and was hesitant about coming into the office alone. She appeared agitated, withdrawn, and distracted. The therapist asked if Lucy could come in while her friend sat in the waiting room, and she agreed.

> Therapist: I can see it was hard for you to enter the office alone, but in spite of that you were able to do it. We need to spend some time this morning talking about what troubles you so that I can be of help.

The therapist does not open the session in the usual manner by asking the patient to describe her problems or what brought her to therapy. The therapist senses that the patient may be seriously impaired and opens the session with support and structure, explaining the therapist's role.

> Lucy: (Haltingly) I don't know what to tell you....My friend thinks I need help. I think I'm falling apart.

The patient responds to the therapist's supportive opening comments and begins to describe what she is experiencing.

> Therapist: Tell me how you think you're falling apart?

Tries to help the patient elaborate and be specific about how she is falling apart.

Lucy: I just sit...I can't get out of bed. I don't want to feed the baby or anything.

Demonstrates that she can be specific and responsive to the therapist. This can be an indicator of the patient's capacity to form a therapeutic alliance.

Therapist: How long has this been going on?

Lucy: Umm...I guess since I found out I was pregnant...but since the baby was born it's worse. I can't stop crying.

The therapist recognizes that the patient may be depressed and focuses on assessing depressive symptomatology and level of functioning. A series of questions are asked to determine whether the patient is depressed and to explore the extent of the depression:

- Are you feeling downhearted? Crying or tearful?
- Are you jumpy, anxious, or agitated?
- Do you feel tired? What is your energy level like?
- Are you able to do your daily tasks at home, at work?
- Have you maintained your social relationships? Do you go out? Does anything give you pleasure?
- Are you having difficulty sleeping or sleeping too much?
- How is your appetite? Are you losing or gaining weight?
- What is your attitude about the future? Do you feel hopeful or hopeless?
- Do you feel life is not worth living? Do you have thoughts of hurting yourself? Suicidal plans? Have you tried to hurt yourself?
- Are you able to have sexual relations? Do you derive pleasure from sex?

Lucy reveals that for the past 4 to 5 weeks she has been consistently agitated, tearful, fatigued, and pessimistic about the future, with thoughts of killing herself, but had no plan. She has difficulty sleeping, waking during the early-morning hours and being unable to get back to sleep. Her appetite is poor, with a weight loss of 15 pounds in the last 3 weeks. She no longer goes out, but remains at home and fails to return telephone calls. A woman from her church is temporarily helping Lucy with the housework and children. Nothing gives Lucy pleasure or satisfaction, and she has no sexual desire or interest. The therapist established that the patient was in the throes of a major depressive episode and went on to inquire about Lucy's past history of depression and related disorders. There were four episodes of major depression, beginning in her early 20s. Between these episodes, Lucy had a chronic low-level depression (double depression) but for the most part was able to care for her daughter and to work.

Therapist: From what you've told me, it seems clear that you're depressed and have had several bouts of depression in the past, but in between these episodes you've been struggling with a milder form of depression that's been with you for much of your life. Let's try to understand how it began this time.

The therapist has begun to educate the patient about her depressive illness. Education is important in all forms of psychotherapy, but especially so in supportive treatment. Education provides the patient with knowledge about his or her difficulties and also demonstrates the therapist's interest in and understanding of the patient and promotes the therapeutic alliance. The therapist then undertakes an exploration of the current episode of depression.

Lucy: Depression...does that mean I'm a mental case, crazy?

Therapist: It means that you're downhearted and have problems that trouble you...that are making you feel so badly about yourself that you can't function in your usual way. You have what is called a depressive illness and have had this several times in your life. It's an illness like any other kind of medical illness, but it doesn't mean crazy. Does that make sense?

Continues the educational process by identifying Lucy's illness and asks for agreement.

Lucy: I guess so. Maybe I'm not crazy, but I can't get John *(her boyfriend)* out of my head. We did things together. He took me places. I wanted to put something positive in my life. My husband and I, we don't do things together, not like husband and wife, we're more like a sister and brother. I keep calling John, but he won't talk to me.

Responds to therapist's explanation and continues to describe her problems with her husband and John.

Therapist: So you've been calling him and he doesn't want to talk with you, that must be rough.

Supportive statements, such as noting that the patient is suffering with depression and commenting on how rough it must be with her boyfriend, constitute supportive trial therapy. These empathic comments were helpful to the patient and enabled her to talk in a meaningful way about the troubles she was having in her relationship. If Lucy had responded negatively to these statements, the therapist might change the technique to one of making contact through listening rather than making empathic statements.

If the patient had little in the way of structural deficits (i.e., was on the right side of the continuum), the therapist might have been more confrontational and asked the patient why she continued to call this abusive boyfriend.

> Lucy: It is *(tearful)*; I like to be with him, we go out and do things that are fun and exciting, otherwise my life is dull and I just go out and walk the street looking for him.

> Therapist: So it's rough in a lot of ways. Not being with John and then you go looking for him *(the therapist restates or clarifies the patient's conflict in an empathic manner)*. What's that like?

> Lucy: It's like, you know, I'm scared.

> Therapist: What does that feel like?

> Lucy: I'm, I don't know, like jumpy, I can't sit still. I keep thinking about him, and then sometimes I start to shake and think I'm going crazy.

The therapist realizes that Lucy is anxious and begins to explore the full extent of her anxiety. The patient went on to describe episodes of panic with somatic concomitants such as shortness of breath, heart pounding, dizziness, lightheadedness, nausea, and fear that she would die or go crazy. Her panic attacks occurred approximately once a week and began 3 years ago. At this point in the interview, it is important for the therapist to obtain information about the panic symptoms and their history rather than continue to explore the relationship with John. As mentioned earlier, exploration of symptoms takes precedence over exploration of relationships, work, or school history.

After investigating the history of the panic, the therapist returned to Lucy's relationship with John. It emerged that the patient was verbally brutalized by John and had no regard for her own safety and well-being. At the same time, Lucy lived with her husband, Carl, who was not abusive but was absent from home a good deal of the time. Carl knew nothing of Lucy's relationship with John. At home, Lucy was barely able to take care of the tasks of daily living, including the care and supervision of her 11-year-old daughter and her infant daughter. Her history revealed many early separations and other traumatic incidents, including severe physical abuse from her mother and neglect from her absent father.

The patient is in the throes of a major depressive episode and has had four previous major depressions as well as a milder chronic depression for most of her life. In addition, she has had panic attacks for the past 3 years. There are serious difficulties in the interpersonal sphere as well as personality problems that limit her ability to function. The therapist, a psychiatrist, concluded that Lucy would benefit from medication and a supportive approach employing cognitive-behavioral techniques. The therapist explained how both approaches—medication and psychotherapy—would be helpful in treating Lucy's depression, anxiety, and problems in day-to-day functioning. The patient was in agreement with these immediate treatment goals and stated that she thought the medication and psychotherapy were worth a try. An explanation was given about when the medication would begin to work and reach its maximum effect, and its possible side effects were discussed.

Case Formulation

Structural Approach

Lucy is an intelligent woman but has limited insight and judgment. Reality testing and adaptation to reality are impaired. She has little regard for her own safety and well-being and is so deeply depressed that she has difficulty functioning.

Her object relations are at a need-satisfying level: others are pursued without regard for their qualities. Lucy has low self-esteem, most likely resulting from both early and current experiences. Her depression has intensified her feelings of inadequacy. She has difficulty forming intimate relationships and tolerating separations. When she is depressed, her ability to be concerned about others becomes impaired, as demonstrated by her difficulty caring for her daughters.

Lucy's defenses are in the immature range, consisting of denial, acting out, and turning against the self. Predominant affects are sadness and anxiety.

Lucy's impaired thinking is reflected in an inability to understand the consequences of her behavior and to think things through in a clear and logical manner. She has many negative thoughts, which will be discussed in the cognitive formulation.

Lucy exhibits little remorse or guilt about her unwillingness to care for her daughters; in addition, she single-mindedly pursues an abusive man while rejecting her husband.

Genetic Approach

Lucy was born to a 16-year-old unmarried mother who left her with a series of caretakers for the first 3 years of life. For the next 2 years, she remained with her mother, a brutal adolescent who was abusive and left her with various caretakers. When Lucy was 5, she was given to her natural father, who was married and had three children. Her stepmother was described as a callous and cold woman who frightened the patient. Her father was away from home a good bit of the time. Lucy cried every night when he was gone, was frightened all the time, and felt that the walls were closing in on her. These traumatic events created problems with normal separation-individuation and attachment. As a child, Lucy was passive, fearful, and depressed. When she was 10 years old, Lucy was returned to her mother, who again repeatedly abandoned her. The repeated abandonments continued into adolescence, a time when teenagers have a second chance to consolidate their identity and resolve separation and oedipal conflicts, and interfered with her ability to develop a cohesive and positive sense of self.

Dynamic Approach

Lucy is a needy, dependent woman who longs for closeness. The central dynamic themes or core conflicts elaborated in the patient's symptomatic acts and character style are her wish to be taken care of and her self-destructive behavior when disappointed by others. The wish to be cared for is an expression of the need to repair feelings of defectiveness, emptiness, and helplessness linked to deprivation, neglect, and brutalization by her mother. Trying to repair the emptiness and loneliness by having a lover satisfies her need for attention and creates a situation in which she is again brutalized. She then engages in self-sabotaging and risk-taking behavior. Lucy seeks relationships with individuals who use, abuse, reject, and neglect her just as her caretakers did when she was a child. She becomes depressed when her tie to the current person in her life becomes problematic. The separation from her abusive boyfriend leads to feelings of worthlessness and craving for closeness at whatever cost. The birth of her second child placed new demands on her, both psychologically and physiologically, at a time when she was extremely needy and was abandoned by John.

Cognitive-Behavioral Approach

Lucy's problems are depression, anxiety, inability to perform the tasks of daily living, and neediness that has resulted in an inappropriate, sadomasochistic extramarital relationship. Her automatic thoughts are "I'm no good; I'm a bad person." These automatic thoughts are derived from Lucy's core beliefs that no one wants her or cares about her, and everyone abandons her. Conditional beliefs are based on the idea that if she is left alone by others, she has no value. Her problematic behavior is to remain with John, demonstrating little frustration tolerance with no regard for the consequences of her actions. The origins of Lucy's core beliefs are the repeated abandonments and abuse by caretaking figures early in life. Precipitants include the birth of her second daughter, her husband's unavailability, and the loss of her boyfriend, all of which increased her need for support. The working hypothesis is that Lucy's depression, anxiety, and neediness are based on the core beliefs that no one wants, cares about, or will sustain her, which were activated by the birth of her daughter, the inattention of her husband, and the loss of her boyfriend. Possible obstacles to treatment include Lucy's considerable neediness, which may create difficulties separating from the therapist and lead to overly compliant behavior.

Diagnostic Evaluation

Axis I	Major depressive disorder, recurrent
	Dysthymic disorder
	Panic disorder
Axis II	Diagnosis deferred (as stated earlier, a personality diagnosis in the presence of a major Axis I diagnosis should be deferred until the patient improves)
Axis III	None
Axis IV	Childbirth and loss of relationship
Axis V	Global Assessment of Functioning (GAF) = 45

Treatment Plan

The treatment plan for this patient is a combined approach using antidepressant medication and supportive psychotherapy. In terms of immediate goals, medication will be used to treat Lucy's mood disturbance and panic attacks, while supportive therapy will be directed at improving her self-esteem, ego functions, and adaptation. Cognitive-behavioral techniques will be used to address Lucy's dysfunctional thinking and thereby ameliorate her depressive symptomatology and negative view of herself.

Initially, efforts will be directed at Lucy's depression and tasks of daily living. As Lucy becomes less depressed and more functional, interpersonal and work issues will be addressed. Ultimate goals include helping the patient return to work and improving her interpersonal relationships. A joint interview with the husband should be planned for further assessment of the patient's difficulties, including the marital relationship.

Session 2

> Therapist: Last week we started to talk about your problems, and you began the medication. Let's continue to try to under-

stand what happened to you and what led to your depression. But before we do that, we need to discuss how you're doing with the medication.

The therapist asks about the medication and focuses on side effects, medication compliance, and dosage adjustment. Whether the therapist is a physician or nonphysician, an exploration of the details surrounding medication should be undertaken. Once this is completed, the therapist inquires about how things have been going since they last met. In so doing, the therapist uses a transitioning process to shift from medication to psychotherapy.

Lucy: I yell at Brenda *(her 11-year-old daughter)*, I'm angry, tired, I don't want to go to work, and I cry all the time...thank God I have someone helping with the baby. John says I cause all his problems—I'm no good, a bad person.

Therapist: He can say what he likes, but that doesn't make it true.

Uses a conversational style and begins to challenge the patient's acceptance of John's negative view of her.

Lucy: I don't know what to think. When he says these things, I believe him. *(Patient is very anxious.)*

Indicates dependence on John and negative thoughts about herself.

Therapist: But if you take a step back and think about it, I mean without your emotions clouding the issue, is it true? What evidence is there that you're a bad person?

Begins the process of a collaborative examination of Lucy's automatic negative thoughts about herself, using an evidenced-based approach.

Lucy: *(Pause)* Oh, I see what you mean...my emotions... get in my way. If I think about it, even though there are things wrong with me, I'm not so bad as John says.

Allows that she may not be as bad as she thought. Therapist wonders if Lucy is being overly compliant by agreeing so readily.

Therapist: Let me clarify...to see if I'm understanding you correctly; at times you don't have a good opinion of yourself, but you think John is wrong, because he goes too far. Don't forget, you've been depressed, and when anyone gets depressed, they tend to think poorly of themselves.

Explains that depression can lead to negative thoughts about the self.

Lucy: Yeah, I get that way. I think I'm no good. I can't do anything...take care of the baby, I cry a lot.

Elaborates on her passivity and negative thoughts.

Therapist: That's the depression in you. It affects how you think
about yourself, and then you begin to think you're no good.

Lucy: Am I going to get out of this?

Therapist: I don't see any reason why not. You've had several episodes of depression in the past and gotten through those.

*Reassures the patient based on the knowledge that the patient has recovered
from previous episodes of depression. The use of reassurance is not indicated
unless the therapist has evidence on which to base the reassurance.*

Lucy: I know what you're saying, but it's hard to remember
that...I still feel I'm no good.

*Returns to negative thoughts about herself. Lucy's earlier agreement was based
on her compliance with therapist.*

Therapist: It may help if we try to think about some positive aspects about you, kind of make a list.

Attempts to shift to constructing evidence for a more positive view of Lucy.

Lucy: Well...I tried to do things for myself.

Therapist: Let's make a list of those things.

Lucy: I started at community college, I like to read...I passed my
courses, but dropped out when I got involved with John.
I only have one semester left and I can graduate, but I can't go
back, I'm just not interested.

Brings up an area of positive functioning from the past.

Therapist: So that's a positive you recognize, you were able to go
to college and pass your courses, but your depression kind
of stopped you. As we know, you've had a problem with self-
esteem most of your life, and the depression makes it worse.

*Clarifies the patient's positive statement and connects it to her problem with
self-esteem.*

> Lucy: Do you mean that like now, I have no confidence and think I am no good?

Attempts to clarify what the therapist has said, much in the same manner as the therapist did earlier. This indicates that the collaborative relationship between the patient and therapist is beginning to develop, since the patient has adopted the therapist's clarifying style.

> Therapist: Yes, because you may, at times, think well of yourself, but when you are in a conflict with John...your emotions take over and you take his word and stop thinking for yourself.

Repeats the same clarification. Repetition is common in all types of psychotherapy and is necessary for the working-through or educational process to be effective.

> Lucy: Yes, I take his word...that's true.

> Therapist: When you get into a conflict with John, it's hard to think well of yourself.

> Lucy: I see that, but I'm so tired and down, it's hard for me to think about these things.

It may be that the therapist has overloaded the patient and she has had enough and is becoming defensive. At this point with this patient, the therapist needs to become more soothing and empathic. On the other hand, in a patient with a more intact structure (i.e., on the right side of the continuum), the therapist might confront the patient's defensive behavior, continuing to work on the conflict or problem.

During this session, the therapist underlined and linked two problems—Lucy's depression and her self-esteem—that will be a focus of treatment. However, the patient also indicated that she has major problems functioning in her everyday life. In the next several sessions, the therapist addressed the patient's everyday functioning, including her care of the children and performance of activities of daily living such as cooking, cleaning, and shopping. In the early phase of treatment, the therapist should help mobilize the patient to assume the tasks of everyday living. Although Lucy has begun antidepressant medication, its effects will not be apparent for several weeks. Therefore, the therapist must be supportive and encouraging until the patient begins to improve and to progress along the continuum.

Session 5

By the fifth session, Lucy had begun to improve. She spoke about her secret fear of being a bad person and cited her behavior during an episode of depression 11 years earlier when she left her daughter alone. At this point, the patient wondered aloud if the therapist really understood her. The therapist suspected that the patient was struggling with the differences between them racially.

Lucy: Do you really know what I mean?

Therapist: So you're asking if I can understand you as a person?

Attempts to clarify Lucy's question.

Lucy: I mean, you're so different from me.

Able to address their differences.

Therapist: Do you mean because I'm a white man and you're an African-American woman? Are you wondering if I can understand you?

Addresses obvious racial and gender differences.

Lucy: Well, I think you understand, but I did so many bad things, like leaving Brenda alone.

Avoids therapist's question.

Therapist: You've been depressed and unable to care for yourself. How could you care for Brenda? You were just too depressed.

Uses explanation to support the reality of Lucy's situation.

Lucy: I guess so.

Therapist: Let's get back to the racial difference between us and the fact that I'm a man and you're a woman. It's important for us to be able to work together comfortably. Have you been feeling uncomfortable with me?

Refocuses Lucy on racial and gender differences.

The therapist used this opportunity to explore Lucy's thoughts and feelings about working with a white male therapist. Cultural differences between patient and therapist, whether racial or ethnic, should routinely be addressed early in treatment and certainly when and if they appear in the material. Gender differences should also be addressed if they become an obstacle to treatment. With Lucy, the therapist postponed raising this issue during the first few sessions because of her depression. By the fifth session, it was the patient who alluded to their differences, enabling the therapist to explore these issues.

Case 2: Supportive-Expressive Psychotherapy— The Woman Who Thought She Was a Murderer

Christine, a 25-year-old secretary, sought treatment 5 months after she was shot three times in the abdomen and critically wounded by her former lover, Tom, who committed suicide after shooting her. Avoidance was Christine's method of handling her troubling symptoms. She hoped that not talking about the devastating attack and Tom's subsequent suicide would help her forget, but nightmares about the shooting and suicide plagued her.

One month after the attempted murder, Christine experienced feelings of despondency, thought she was falling apart and losing control of her mind. She felt estranged from the world, anesthetized, and disoriented. Both the events leading up to the attempted murder and suicide and their aftermath were recreated in her mind like a movie endlessly repeating itself. Christine was unable to stop sobbing. Facing her friends and her ex-boyfriends' family was impossible, since she felt guilty about his death and was deeply ashamed.

The patient is the oldest of three children. She has two brothers, 1 and 3 years her junior, who were favored by her parents. Her parents have a conflictual relationship that Christine traces to her conception, which occurred prior to their marriage. She was referred to as "the accident." Her father, an alcoholic, is both physically and verbally abusive to all members of the family. Christine's mother is a depressed, withdrawn, dependent woman who is passive and ineffectual. Christine's brothers, like Christine, have conflictual relationships with both parents.

Session 1

At the first session, Christine reluctantly spoke about the death of her boyfriend, Tom.

Therapist: Can you tell me what the problem is?

Christine: (*She is reticent and speaks haltingly*) I feel...respon-
sible...for Tom's death....I could have prevented it. I can't
get it out...of my mind.

Therapist: Can you tell me what happened?

Asks for specifics.

Christine: Tom shot himself in the head. He killed himself.

Therapist: My God!

Empathic exclamation and spontaneous reaction.

Christine: He drove away, leaving me on the ground.

Responds to therapist's exclamation.

Therapist: He left you on the ground? How did that happen?

*Recognizes Christine's difficulty speaking about the events surrounding the
shooting, but continues to explore what happened to learn about the patient and
to determine the appropriate type of psychotherapy.*

Christine: Yes,...he...shot me before he drove away.

Therapist: He shot you?

*The response of disbelief and amazement may be perceived negatively by the
patient and can interfere with the alliance.*

Christine: Three times, twice in the car and once when I was on
the ground.

The patient hesitantly described being dragged into Tom's car when
she was returning from work. He was in a frenzied state, shrieking that she
was a whore and unfaithful to him. He stopped the car and shot her twice
in the abdomen. Somehow she managed to escape from the car and crawled
onto the sidewalk, where he shot her one more, then drove away and fatally
shot himself. Christine's emphasis when recounting these events was on
Tom's suicide.

Therapist: From what you've told me about being shot three
times, you must have been severely injured, yet you minimize what happened to you.

Addresses defensive minimization.

Christine: Well...I feel terrible about Tom.

Continues to be defensive, suppressing her needs.

Therapist: And you, were you seriously injured?

Maintains focus on patient and her injuries.

Christine: I almost died. I was rushed to the hospital and had emergency surgery. I was a mess. The doctors told my mother that they didn't know if I would pull through. I lost a lot of blood. Look!!! (*Patient lifts her blouse, revealing scars across her abdomen extending to her back.*)

Therapist: What a harrowing experience it must have been for you. I can see how hard it is to talk about it, because it causes you such anguish even now, but it's important that we continue to talk about it so that we can understand what happened to you and help you come to grips with these difficult feelings and experiences.

Offers an empathic comment coupled with an explanation of how therapy might help.

Christine: I should have died. (*Begins to cry and becomes more anxious.*) I can't believe it happened.

Returns to feelings of guilt.

Therapist: What makes you think you should have died?

Begins to explore her guilt.

Christine: I left him and was dating another guy. If I hadn't done that, he wouldn't have gotten so angry at me. He wouldn't have killed himself.

Dysfunctional thinking.

Therapist: You feel responsible for Tom's death despite the fact that he pulled the trigger.

Addresses dysfunctional thinking.

Christine: Yes (*becomes visibly anxious*), I know, but I can't talk about it (*begins to cry*).

Talking about the events that occurred increased rather than diminished the patient's anxiety. Confronting the patient with her avoidant behavior and pressing for more details of the attack evoked the symptoms that were most troubling to Christine. The therapist became more supportive, no longer confronting the patient when she became avoidant, and gathered the following additional history.

The patient had been in a chaotic, abusive relationship with Tom for 7 years. They met when she was 15 years old and parted many times during the subsequent years. She indicated that she got nothing from the relationship—they watched television and fought a lot. At times he beat her. Although she wanted to live with him, he refused to allow her to move into his apartment, yet expected her to be available whenever he called. Six months prior to the shooting, Christine had ended the relationship. Since that time, Tom had prohibited her from socializing with friends. At first she went along with his wish, because she was afraid of him, but eventually she began to date others. As Christine described these events to the therapist, she was cautious, watchful, and reticent.

During the first interview, the therapist learned that Christine had severe anxiety, depression, and nightmares. Her anxiety was diffuse and generalized and her depression moderately severe. She had difficulty sleeping and was frequently awakened by nightmares, and her concentration was impaired. Christine was not suicidal, but she had flashbacks of Tom shooting her and often had images of his suicide. Focusing on Tom' suicide, she avoided acknowledging the life-threatening situation she had been in, became detached from her friends, and showed little interest in her usual activities. Christine also felt guilty about and responsible for Tom's death. The patient had not been able to mourn for Tom, nor had she allowed herself to feel much about her own victimization and long-term abuse, both physical and verbal. She worried about her future and wondered if she would ever get married or have children.

Patient and therapist discussed the goals of treatment and agreed on the immediate and ultimate aims (see Treatment Plan below for a description of specific goals).

Case Formulation

Structural Approach

Christine is a woman of average intelligence with only superficial insight into her difficulties. Her reality testing is generally intact, but her judgment and adaptation to reality are faulty, as evidenced by her remaining in an abusive relationship with her boyfriend. Although unable to work at present, Christine had been responsible and conscientious in her job prior to the shooting.

The patient's dependency and fear of separation and loss interfere with the quality of her relationships, resulting in impaired object relations. She has a long history of passively submitting to a physically abusive, highly conflictual, and demeaning relationship. Christine tends to set aside her own needs, giving priority to the wishes and needs of others at her own expense. Her low self-esteem is reflected in her readiness to accept blame; both her own and the anticipated harsh judgment of others. Her predominant affects are depression and guilt. Christine denies anger about being shot but torments herself with excessive feelings of guilt about Tom's death. Major defenses used are denial, avoidance, rationalization, and helplessness. The patient's inability to endure object loss affects her frustration tolerance and capacity to delay gratification.

In general, Christine's synthetic functioning is uneven. Although she performs well at work, in her intimate and social relationships there is considerable chaos. In terms of morals, ideals, and conscience (superego), Christine is harshly critical of herself and experiences excessive guilt.

Genetic Approach

As a young child, Christine felt unwanted by her parents, who favored her younger brothers. Conceived prior to their hastily arranged marriage, Christine described her parents as immature, argumentative, and critical. Her father, an alcoholic, was remote, unavailable, and physically abusive. Her mother, a depressed woman, became pregnant when the patient was 3 months old, thus placing an additional burden on her limited emotional resources. She was passive and unable to protect Christine from her father's abusive behavior. The repetitive nature of her mother's neglect, coupled with physical abuse from her father, affected Christine's ability to develop a sense of self with value and contributed to a negative self-image and poor object choices.

Dynamic Approach

The patient is struggling with ambivalent feelings toward her dead boyfriend. Christine has the fantasy of being a murderer and feels guilty and sad, blaming herself for Tom's suicide while denying angry feelings toward him for attempting to kill her. Ambivalence also characterizes Christine's conflicts with her father. She hides her anger and disappointment with him by making excuses for his behavior and lack of interest in her welfare. Christine's relationship with her mother is somewhat better, but unsatisfying. She longs for a close, caring relationship with both mother and father, but holds back, fearing rejection from her father and withdrawal from her mother. According to the core conflictual relationship theme (CCRT) model, Christine's wish (W) is to be loved or cared for, and the response of the other (R_O) is abuse, hostility, criticism, and disinterest. Christine's own current response (R_S) is anxiety and depression, while maintaining her characteristic behavior of attempting to please others.

Cognitive-Behavioral Approach

Christine's problems are anxiety, depression, flashbacks to the traumatic incident, and an inability to return to work and face other people. Her thinking is fraught with automatic thoughts such as "I left Tom, so he killed himself, and I'm responsible for his death" and "Tom was nasty to me because I wasn't nice enough to him." Core beliefs include a sense of not being good enough or wanted. Her conditional beliefs are that 1) if she had been better to Tom, he would not have shot her or killed himself; and 2) unless she is totally submissive, she is no good and will not be loved by anyone. The origins of Christine's core beliefs are her early experiences of feeling unwanted, being physically abused by her father, and feeling unprotected by her withdrawn mother. The activating situation was Tom's shooting of Christine and his suicide. The working hypothesis is that Christine's anxiety, depression, flashbacks, and guilt are based on her core belief that she is not good enough, which was activated by the shooting. Possible obstacles include Christine's wish to please the therapist and her tendency to avoid her true thoughts and feelings in treatment.

Diagnostic Evaluation

Axis I	Posttraumatic stress disorder
Axis II	Diagnosis deferred
Axis III	Postsurgery from gunshot wounds
Axis IV	Suicide of boyfriend and his attempted murder of her
Axis V	GAF = 50

Treatment Plan

The psychotherapy of patients with posttraumatic stress disorder has evolved considerably. In the past, many patients who suffered from this disorder were immediately confronted with the traumatic event or situation, and some patients became destabilized, which created difficulties in their treatment. As always, a flexible approach should be designed that gauges the patient's ability to work on the traumatic event. Many individuals cannot immediately explore the trauma, but instead may require support and the forging of a collaborative therapeutic relationship.

For Christine, a supportive approach to promote stability will be used initially, because she appeared to be unable to continue the exploration of her traumatic experience during the evaluation interview. The first few sessions will be devoted to helping Christine with her interpersonal relationships, self-esteem, dysfunctional thinking, and preparation for return to work. As the patient's equilibrium returns and the therapeutic alliance becomes secure, exposure therapy (see Chapter 5) will be used. Christine then can be encouraged to talk about the traumatic event so that it can be reexperienced in a controlled setting without overwhelming anxiety. Exposure therapy will enable Christine to become desensitized to the trauma and to work through the thoughts and feelings associated with it. Finally, Christine's core conflict—her wish to be loved and cared for, which results in her attempts to please others, often at a tremendous cost to herself—must be explored and worked through. Accordingly, the immediate goals of treatment are to restore Christine's equilibrium by diminishing the symptoms of posttraumatic stress disorder and enhancing her self-esteem. Ultimate goals of treatment are to improve object relations so that the patient can make better choices about the men in her life, separate from her parents, and return to work.

Session 4

Christine entered the therapist's office appearing sad, sat down, and looked at the therapist expectantly.

Therapist: Is something troubling you?

The therapist actively attempts to engage the patient. With more structurally intact patients (i.e., those on the right side of the continuum), it is preferable to wait for the patient to begin. This enables the therapist to more readily recognize the adaptive context.

Christine: Well... I've been having trouble with my parents. They say all I do is mope around. They want me to start living my life... you know, to get back to work.

Indicates problem.

Therapist: What's that like for you?

Christine: I feel pushed, like pressured.

Therapist: So your parents are pushing you....

Clarifies to help patient elaborate.

Christine: I don't like it when they push at me, especially my father. He's a rough customer. He gets nasty when there's trouble.

Focuses more specifically on father.

Therapist: Did something happen recently with your father? Can you give me an example?

Asks for specific example.

Christine: I think it was 2 days ago...he came home from work and found me watching television. He got annoyed and said, "What are you doing home? Get yourself back to work! You just lazy around all day...I'm not going to support you forever." *(Ends in tears.)*

Therapist: That must have been upsetting. How did you handle it?

Responds with empathy and asks for a behavior rather than a feeling. The patient is overwhelmed with feelings and has trouble responding to her feelings.

Christine: I turned off the television, went to my room and cried.

Indicates maladaptive response.

Therapist: So when he's nasty, you become teary and run away. Have you thought of any other ways of dealing with your father?

Clarifies and engages patient to consider other coping strategies.

Christine: When I talk back and get mad it's even worse; even at my age he'd slam me. That's what he does with my mother.

Indicates that the alternative strategy of standing up to father can be dangerous.

Therapist: With your father you think you're trapped. If you stand up for yourself he'll get more brutal, and if you do nothing you think you're helpless and defeated.

Summarizes patient's dilemma.

> Christine: That's right.

> Therapist: Are there only two choices? What alternatives can we
> come up with?

Indicates that patient polarizes her choices into two unacceptable alternatives.
Suggests a collaborative problem-solving approach.

> Christine: I could kill him *(laughs)*.

A fantasy emerges in the guise of a joke.

> Therapist: Well that's one choice, any others?

Continues to focus on choices.

> Christine: Well if my mother had left him years ago, that would
> have helped.

Blames mother while taking a passive stance.

> Therapist: Is that a choice for you?

Suggests possible choice involving an active role.

> Christine: I have thought of moving out, but I can't afford it.
> I would have to go back to work.

> Therapist: Well, have you thought about that?

Continues to help patient problem-solve.

> Christine: I want to go back…but I can't face the others at my
> job.

Raises new concern.

> Therapist: How come?

> Christine: I don't know what they think of me.

Reflects negative thoughts about herself.

Therapist: What do you think is on their minds?

Explores.

Christine: That I'm responsible for my boyfriend's death.

Automatic thought projected onto others. Christine casts herself as a murderer. Relationship to joke about murdering her father?

Therapist: Why would anyone think that? You didn't shoot him.

Reality-tests and reassures.

Christine: No, I didn't. You know, before the shooting I was going to move out to my own apartment...I mean share one with my friend Amy, but since Tom died, I haven't been able to do anything.

Moves into problem-solving mode and positive alliance.

Therapist: Yes...well, you needed time to recover from your injuries and surgery. Do you feel stronger now—strong enough to begin planning again?

Checks to see if patient is ready to move ahead.

Christine: I think I do. I just hate to be pushed.

Agrees to go ahead but indicates that perhaps the therapist is experienced like father.

Therapist: Do you think that we're going too fast...that I'm pushing you, sort of the way your father does?

Links self with father (transference interpretation).

Christine: No...no, you're nothing like my father.

Denies connection.

Therapist: I know you want to pull things together in your life, but I don't want you to feel pushed by me. You've been through a rough time.

Therapist acknowledges error.

> Christine: You know, I forgot to tell you that my boss called me a few days ago. He wants me to come back to work. What do you think?

Continues to work collaboratively after therapist acknowledges error.

> Therapist: You said that it would be hard for you to face your co-workers, so we need to talk about that. But since your boss called, he must be interested and concerned about you. Do you think that's true?

Begins to support self-esteem.

> Christine: He wants me back...I know that, but what will I say to the other people at work?

> Therapist: Let's play that out...as if I'm one of your co-workers. Okay?

The therapist has initiated a role-playing exercise to prepare the patient for encounters with others. This will help her respond to their questions and comments and achieve a sense of mastery over encounters of this sort.

Two weeks later, the patient returned to work on a part-time basis. The therapist continued to be supportive while beginning to explore Christine's difficulties at work and with her parents. She was asked to keep a journal listing her automatic negative thoughts (e.g., "Others will blame me for Tom's death"; "I'm a bad person"). It was not until the midphase (Session 5) of treatment that an in-depth exploration of the shootings was undertaken.

Case 3: Expressive-Supportive Psychotherapy— Sarah's Choice

Sarah, a 65-year-old married woman with two grown sons, entered treatment because she felt depressed and pessimistic about the future. Seven months prior to seeking treatment, the patient had failed to get an anticipated promotion at work, learned that her older son was planning to get married and move to a distant state, and discovered that her husband was considering retiring.

A salient factor in this patient's past is that she is a concentration camp survivor. Sarah's mother, father, grandmother, and two sisters were all murdered in the concentration camp. Sarah acknowledged that for 40 years she has hidden everything that had happened to her because she didn't want anyone, including her family, to pity her.

Session 1

> Therapist: Tell me about what's troubling you.

The evaluation begins with a rapid survey of problems. With this in mind, the therapist pursues each area of disturbance thoroughly.

> Sarah: Dr. Goodrich (the patient's internist) suggested that I come to see you. I told him I'm having a nervous breakdown.

Presents a general statement.

> Therapist: Can you describe what that has been like?

Asks for details.

> Sarah: A black mood.

Offers a bit more, but is terse and does not volunteer information.

> Therapist: A black mood; do you feel that way right now?

Brings problem into the here and now to make the problem come alive and to be more immediate.

> Sarah: Yes, I'm useless, I've been dumped (irritated).

Acknowledges her feeling in the moment, but does not give details.

> Therapist: Tell me more about the black mood.

Holds Sarah to describing black mood.

> Sarah: Nothing is good in my life...and I don't expect anything in the future.

> Therapist: Are you feeling downhearted?

> Sarah: Yes, I am, but I do what I have to do.

The therapist inquires about symptoms of depression such as sleep, appetite, energy level, and suicidal feelings. It is preferable to explore symptoms before relationship and characterological factors (see Chapter 3). Sarah indicates that she has no problems in these areas, but is generally pessimistic and irritable (black mood). She reports that her black mood became worse recently when she had a problem at work.

> Therapist: Tell me what happened at work to make your black mood worse.

> Sarah: I was in line for a promotion, and my supervisor—she neglected to send in the necessary papers recommending me, so it was given to someone else. This other woman isn't as good at the job as I am, even though I was there only 6 months.

> Therapist: Your supervisor was neglectful and didn't go to bat for you. What's her name?

Clarifies and then asks for the supervisor's name. Asking the patient for specifics regarding people mentioned helps promote relatedness to others and adds to the liveliness of the interaction between patient and therapist.

> Sarah: Doreen; she didn't care about my promotion.

> Therapist: What were you feeling toward Doreen?

> Sarah: Furious...I...so I quit, walked out. I thought...this is giving me a nervous breakdown.

Readily declares her anger.

> Therapist: So you were furious at Doreen; is that what made you feel as if you were having a nervous breakdown?

> Sarah: Yes; no one cares about me.

In the initial interview, the therapist should obtain an overview or survey of the patient's most troubling problems. This survey should be relatively brief and should be followed by a return to each area in greater depth. A brief description of this problem area having been elicited, the therapist turned to other difficulties in Sarah's life.

> Therapist: So if I understand you correctly, you were furious at Doreen because she neglected you. We'll get back to this in greater detail in a little while, but are there any other significant problems in your life?

Sarah: I have had thoughts of separating from my husband...but I'm from the old school, where when you make a commitment, you stick to it.

Presents conflict.

Therapist: What is your relationship like with your husband? What's your husband's first name?

Sarah: Ernest; we met at a social for displaced persons. I seem to draw people to me, but then I don't hang on to them for long. My husband and I, we had similar experiences. I hate men...if I had to do it all again, I would never get married. I resent Ernest. He expects me to serve him, to take care of the woman's duties. It's not me that's important, but what he can get out of me.

Presents more information than previously as she discusses her anger toward Ernest.

Therapist: Can you give me an example of how it is between the two of you?

Asks for specific example.

Sarah: He doesn't talk to me, he just expects me to prepare his dinner and clean up. A few days ago, the insurance agent came to the house. I've known him for years, but my husband told me they had business to discuss, so I should leave them alone. I was furious. Later, after the insurance agent left, I told my husband how angry I was, but he thinks I'm crazy and have no reason to be angry.

Presents herself as a victim.

Therapist: So after dinner you expected to be part of the rest of the evening and were excluded by Ernest. Is that what generally happens between the two of you?

Clarifies.

The therapist goes on to complete the survey by asking what other major problems the patient is confronting. Sarah acknowledges that she is troubled because her older son, Steven, will be getting married in 6 months and moving to another state some distance away.

This completes the brief survey of the areas of difficulty in the patient's life. The therapist then returns to the problem with Sarah's supervisor in greater detail.

Therapist: Now that we've briefly gone over your major concerns let's go back to talking about what happened between you and Doreen. You told me you were furious with her for not recommending you for promotion. What did the fury to-ward Doreen feel like inside you?

Begins inquiry using triangles of conflict and person (see Chapter 3). Focuses on Sarah's inner experience of the feeling toward Doreen.

Sarah: I had been on the job for 6 months, it was okay, but there was no feedback from Doreen. She never said I was doing a good job...no one worked as efficiently or quickly as I did. Sometimes I made mistakes, the same one three times over, but there was no one to explain how to do it right.

Gives important information, but avoids talking about her feelings toward Doreen.

Therapist: What you're saying is important and we'll return to that, but you seem to be avoiding your angry feelings toward Doreen.

Confronts Sarah's defensive avoidance.

Sarah: She didn't treat me right, didn't try to help me at all.

Remains at the defensive corner of the triangle of conflict.

Therapist: I can see how hard it is for you to talk about your angry feelings, but it's important for us to understand what was go-ing on inside you and how you felt the anger toward Doreen.

Empathic confrontation of avoidance.

Sarah: I was angry, so angry that I felt blinded, like I couldn't see.

Able to give inner experience of anger.

Therapist: What else were you experiencing inside yourself?

Sarah: Well...it was like a choking in my throat as if it was going to burst apart, I felt the fury pouring out. I had to get away from her...so I quit the job.

At this point, Sarah is able to describe the inner experience and phys-iological manifestations of her anger in a clear and direct manner without being avoidant. Thus far, trial therapy has demonstrated that the patient can tolerate confrontation and express feelings, suggesting her suitability for expressive psychotherapy (i.e., right side of the continuum).

> Therapist: So it started with blinding anger and a choking sensation in your throat. If you let yourself go in your mind, with Doreen, how would it have gone?

Asks for the third part of an affective experience, the fantasy. The other components are the inner experience, including the physiological state and motoric manifestations.

> Sarah: You mean like what I wanted to do to her?

> Therapist: Yes, what did you want to do to Doreen?

> Sarah: I wanted to shout at her and tell her that she doesn't know how to do her job. I couldn't talk to her. She didn't care. She didn't seem to know I was doing a good job.

Relates fantasy, but in reality withdrew without standing up for herself.

> Therapist: You were furious at Doreen and had the wish to shout at her, but instead you withdrew.

Summarizes (clarifies) her active wish and defensive withdrawal.

> Sarah: I knew it wouldn't do any good, she didn't care about me.

Expresses resignation and defensively withdraws.

> Therapist: In a sense, you were left on your own, and in spite of that, you managed to do a good job, but Doreen didn't recognize your work. Could it be that at first you were disappointed in Doreen and then became angry or furious and thought that meant you were "having a nervous breakdown"?

Supportively praises and then reframes the meaning of the "nervous breakdown."

> Sarah: Oh, well...yes, that may be right. I did feel disappointed. But what could I do? She could have written the recommendation. I thought she had. I thought she liked my work.

States she was victimized by Doreen, but acknowledges feeling disappointed and then unable to assert herself in an adaptive manner.

Therapist: You thought Doreen liked your work and maybe you too, so when she disappointed you, you became furious at her and then quit your job. It was hard for you to stand up to her, so you ended up sabotaging yourself.

Sarah: I couldn't stay after that; it was like she dumped me.

Therapist: But what seems to have occurred is that you didn't get dumped, you dumped Doreen and your job after you became disappointed and furious, in a way you sabotaged yourself, do you agree?

Confronts Sarah's self-sabotage and corrects her cognitive distortion that Doreen dumped her.

Sarah: (*Thoughtfully*) I dumped Doreen...yes, you could say that. I felt badly, treated like a nothing, I was unhappy, so I quit!

Accepts reframing.

Therapist: You were in pain because of what happened between you and Doreen, and you reacted by quitting your job and running away.

Sarah: Yes, I couldn't bear to be near Doreen anymore...it was too upsetting.

The therapist's interpretation is part of a trial therapy that tests the patient's ability to tolerate exploration of her wishes, affects, and defenses. Through use of the interventions described above, the patient's ability to observe her behavior and work in therapy was established.

This part of the interview can be understood by applying the triangles of conflict and person. Notice that Doreen is a current person in the patient's life in the triangle of the person. Sarah's wish or need for recognition from Doreen can be viewed from within the triangle of conflict at the wish, need, or feeling corner of the triangle. When Doreen neglected to recommend her for a promotion, Sarah was sad and disappointed at first, then became furious. Her fury created feelings of fear/anxiety (anxiety corner of triangle of conflict), leading to a sense that she would "break down," so she quit her job. Sarah used avoidance (defense corner of triangle of conflict) of her feelings and thought of herself as a victim (helpless stance). Quitting was a maladaptive self-sabotaging defense—an attempt to deal with the intolerable affects of disappointment and anger. In addition, her cognitive distortion of being dumped was addressed.

In this initial interview, the therapist continued to explore the patient's relationships with her family and historical data regarding her early life and adolescent years. Sarah is Jewish and a Holocaust survivor. She is a bitter, somewhat depressed woman who feels useless, superfluous, unwanted, and uncared for. She has been married for 35 years to a man who is 9 years her senior and also a Holocaust survivor. She expresses anger toward her husband for dominating her and has thought of separation many times during their marriage, but is resigned to remaining with him. In general, she dislikes men, including her husband, stating that they make slaves out of women, who have to serve them in every way possible.

Case Formulation

Structural Approach

The area of object relations is most problematic for this patient. Her sense of self is somewhat unstable and characterized by grandiosity alternating with self-deprecation. Sarah devalues others, yet tries to accommodate to their wishes. Others are experienced as withholding, critical, unappreciative, and unavailable. She keeps her distance and maintains only casual social relationships. Despite these problems, she has achieved object constancy.

Although impulse control is generally satisfactory, when frustrated, she impulsively makes decisions that are self-sabotaging, such as suddenly quitting her job. Sarah's predominant affects are anger, irritation, and sadness.

The defenses used are externalization, projection, avoidance, and displacement. The behavioral manifestations of these defenses are blaming, evasion, and being highly critical of others.

Sarah's relation to reality is basically intact, except for her adaptation to reality, which is vulnerable to regression in stressful situations. When Sarah acts impulsively, she gets into difficulties in her everyday life.

Genetic Approach

Sarah was born in Eastern Europe and is the oldest of three sisters. She was considered to be the capable but plain child, while her sisters were characterized as intelligent, pretty, and lovable. As a young child, Sarah was jealous and resentful of her two younger sisters and believed that her parents preferred and admired them. Her mother was experienced as cold and disapproving and she in turn felt unappreciated and afraid of her mother's criticism. Her father, although portrayed as admiring of her, was away for long periods of time. Between the ages of 3 and 7, when her father was away on business, the patient slept with her mother. When her father returned from his travels, Sarah was sent to her own bed. At those times, she felt angry with her father and rejected by her mother. At the same time she felt the need to anticipate her parents' needs and wishes and to comply with them.

When Sarah was 14 years old, she and her family were sent to a concentration camp, where the entire family was exterminated. During the selection process, against her mother's wishes, Sarah chose to join other teenage girls and leave her family. This act of independence saved Sarah's life, because those sent to a work detail had a better chance of survival. Throughout her life she has felt guilty about abandoning her family and surviving. Sarah has never completely mourned the loss of her family. After the war, she wandered about Eastern Europe and spent time in a camp for displaced persons. She came to the United States at age 19.

Dynamic Approach

The central conflict in the patient's life is her wish (W) for admiration and love from others. When others respond with indifference or rejection (R_O), Sarah's response is disappointment, anger, withdrawal, loss of self-esteem, and self-sabotage. A recent example of this was when Sarah impulsively quit her job after she was passed over for a promotion. Historically, this is related to her wish to be preferred by her mother and father. When her father returned from his travels, she was furious at him and her mother for excluding her from the parental bed. Sarah suffers from pathological mourning in relation to her mother, father, and sisters. Anger directed at her husband is used to distance him, protecting her from painful wishes to be loved and admired. The patient feels guilty about her anger toward her parents and believes she deserves to be punished for these feelings. Sarah anticipates losing her son when he gets married and moves to a distant state. This conflict is related to her multiple losses as an adolescent.

Cognitive-Behavioral Approach

The problem list includes anger, self-sabotage, a conflictual relationship with her husband, and vulnerability to loss. Sarah's automatic thoughts are "I am not valued by others" and "life is stacked against me." These automatic thoughts are based on the core belief that she doesn't measure up to others and will be ignored or rejected.

The origins of her core beliefs are early experiences in which Sarah felt she had fewer positive attributes than her sisters. She experienced her parents as rejecting and interpreted her separation from them in the concentration camp as an abandonment and rejection.

The working hypothesis is that Sarah's anger and feelings of vulnerability are based on her belief that she doesn't measure up to others and will be rejected. This was activated by her supervisor's promotion of another employee and not selecting the patient, conflict with her husband associated with his retirement, and her son's impending marriage.

Obstacles to treatment include the possibility of a rupture in the therapeutic alliance as result of Sarah's disdain for others, vulnerability, anger, and impulsivity.

Diagnostic Evaluation

Axis I	Adjustment disorder with depressed mood and pathological mourning
Axis II	Personality disorder not otherwise specified (NOS) with narcissistic and impulsive features
Axis III	None
Axis IV	Passed over for promotion, marital problems, and impending marriage of son
Axis V	GAF = 70

Treatment Plan

During the evaluation and trial therapy, Sarah responded meaningfully to interventions such as confrontation and interpretation. She was able to experience strong affects, including anger, sorrow, and guilt. The treatment approach chosen for this patient was an expressive one with supportive elements, which places her on the right side of the continuum. The decision to use some supportive techniques is based on the structural assessment, which revealed the patient's tendency to both undervalue and overvalue herself; therefore, particular attention will be given to issues of self-esteem. Cognitive approaches will be used to address her negative view of herself and others. The initial focus of treatment will be an exploration of Sarah's pathological mourning and how it affects her current life. Once her pathological mourning or grief is worked through, therapy can be directed toward an exploration of conflicts with her husband, boss, son, and the therapist, and the role of past experiences and fantasies in her current life. The goals of treatment are the facilitation and resolution of the mourning process and the integration of the affective and cognitive aspects of her life, which in turn should enhance Sarah's self-esteem, enable her to return to work, and allow her to resolve conflicts about her husband and son.

Session 4

Sarah entered the therapist's office in a brisk, don't-bother-me manner. She sat down silently and did not make eye contact.

> Therapist: You're silent; is something on your mind?

Confronts silence.

> Sarah: Ernest is impossible (*said in exasperated manner*). He sits down at the table with his fork in his hand and asks, "Is it ready?" I'm always ready. He exasperates me. I just started to look for a new job, but he doesn't want me to do anything, just take care of him. He doesn't like it that I come here, and he bothers me about the insurance and getting the forms done. I'm tired of it all. I just can't do it.

The adaptive context appears to relate to her sense of being exasperated by Ernest and the inference that she may have ambivalent feelings toward the therapist.

> Therapist: What are you experiencing toward Ernest?

Explores feelings toward Ernest and postpones examination of the patient-therapist relationship.

> Sarah: It's too much pressure from Ernest. He doesn't make me feel good.

Vague response, but may be an allusion to the therapist.

> Therapist: How is that?

Maintains focus.

> Sarah: I told you already (*with annoyance*), he doesn't admire me or say anything nice to me. He complains about me and says critical things to our sons. I'm the one with the problems... not him.

Reveals irritation toward therapist and Ernest.

> Therapist: So Ernest doesn't like you to come to see me. How do you feel about seeing me?

Addresses Sarah's feeling toward therapist.

> Sarah: It's fine.

Denies feeling.

> Therapist: I may be wrong, but you seem irritated with me.

Persists with exploration of Sarah's anger by supplying the feeling, but couching it as a speculation.

> Sarah: (*Silence*) In the beginning I thought it would be nice, you seemed to understand me, like Dr. Davis (previous therapist) did. He thought I was terrific; he always said that I managed so well. (*She looks brighter, less irritated, even flirtatious and somewhat seductive.*)

Compares therapist unfavorably with former therapist.

> Therapist: So Dr. Davis admired you and made you feel terrific.... Can you tell me what it's like for you to be here with me? — because you do seem irritated.

Clarifies, then holds Sarah to her feelings toward therapist.

> Sarah: It makes me uneasy. He used to reassure me.

Expresses anxiety about not being reassured.

> Therapist: So you feel uneasy about your irritation with me. Tell me about feeling uneasy.

The therapist is working within the triangle of conflict by noting the patient's uneasiness, indicating that she is experiencing anxiety in reaction to her irritation with the therapist.

> Sarah: I'm unsure. You don't reassure me...I feel apprehensive.

Confirms that anxiety is related to not being reassured.

> Therapist: So you're experiencing apprehension or anxiety in relation to the irritation you feel toward me. How do you experience the irritation toward me?

> Sarah: I don't know.

Defensive helplessness.

> Therapist: You say you don't know, sort of making yourself helpless. It's important that we get to talk about and understand your thoughts and feelings.

Confronts defensive helplessness and underlines the importance of getting to Sarah's feelings.

> Sarah: I'm not used to telling what I feel.

Oppositional avoidance.

> Therapist: I know it's hard for you to talk to me so directly about your feelings, but you're avoiding them with me just as you always have.

Confronts Sarah's avoidance.

> Sarah: Yes, well, I am angry with you. I don't know how to be with you, you don't reassure me.

Declares anger toward therapist.

> Therapist: So you're angry with me for not reassuring you as Dr. Davis did.

Clarifies anger toward therapist for not satisfying her need to be reassured.

> Sarah: Yes.

> Therapist: I think there may be times you won't feel immediately reassured by me. Sometimes it's more important to get to what you're really feeling inside yourself.

The therapist does not explore Sarah's inner experience of anger, but instead chooses to be more supportive by offering an explanation of how therapy works. The therapist might have continued to test Sarah's ability to respond to a more challenging approach. However, at that moment it appeared that the therapeutic alliance was problematic, and the therapist attempted to repair it by shifting to a more supportive approach.

> Sarah: (*Pause*) You're courageous to say that to me. No one has spoken to me so directly since I lost my parents. I don't understand what's happening, but I don't want to stir up a hornet's nest. Don't take it personally, but I don't want you to waste your energy. I always wanted to anticipate what people wanted, always wanted to please.

Responds to therapist's explanation and indicates she habitually wants to please.

> Therapist: How is that with me?

Explores need to please within the patient-therapist relationship.

> Sarah: *(Silence)*...It was my birthday last week, and Dr. Davis called to wish me happy birthday.... I found out all about his personal life. My time with him was like a social hour, he commiserated with me. I don't know what you want or how to be with you.

Expresses wish for a more personal relationship with therapist.

> Therapist: How do you imagine I want you to be?

Asks for fantasy.

> Sarah: Well...my mother always taught me not to take anything from anyone. There was a woman who lived not too far away from us. She baked the most wonderful cookies. Her house always smelled good, and I loved to visit. I knew she baked such wonderful cookies because several times she brought them to my house, but I was not allowed to have any of them when we visited her house. "Do not act like you want them," my mother would caution me. One Saturday my parents, my younger sister, and I went to visit. She brought out a plate of her cookies and passed them around. The adults helped themselves; I said, "No, thank you," and so did my sister. Sometime later she passed the cookies around again; I was longing for them, but I said, "No, thank you." When she passed them to my sister, she said, "No, thank you...but if you ask me again, I will say yes." Everyone laughed and she was given two cookies, which she immediately ate.

Reveals she was taught by her mother not to ask for what she wants.

> Therapist: You tried to go along with your mother's wishes. It's the same with me; wanting me to be interested and care about you, so you attempt to please me and then get irritated with me if you think I'm not caring the way Dr. Davis was.

Brings together the triangle of conflict and triangle of the person by linking Sarah's conflict with the therapist to a similar conflict with her mother.

The session continued with further exploration of Sarah's relationship with her mother.

> Sarah: I think I became rebellious when I was going on 14. I wanted to find my way. *(She became softer and her eyes filled*

with tears.) Maybe I was obnoxious sometimes. I was almost 14 when we went to the concentration camp—my mother, father, grandmother, and my sisters. There were two groups. It was up to me to choose...I wanted to be with the older girls. My mother tried to hold me with her, but I ran over to the older group. My mother told the commander, "She's only 13." She wanted me to be with her. Why didn't she...force me to stay with her or come with me? My grandmother could have stayed with my sisters.

Indicates that she had rebelled against mother, but wishes mother had held on to her.

Therapist: You said no to your mother and never saw her again.

Connects saying no to mother to losing her.

Sarah: *(long pause)*...I wanted to show her I could do what I want. She was a very strong woman.

Therapist: But then you lost her.

Links independence with losing mother.

Sarah: Why didn't she force me to go? She should have forced me.

Expresses anguish about mother's powerlessness.

Therapist: Saying no to your mother saved your life...you were an adolescent then and wanting independence. Saying no to me may seem like the safer way, but you don't have to run away from me to save your life.

The therapist recognized Sarah's wish to get away from treatment when she spoke of Ernest wanting her to stop, and connected this wish to leaving her mother when she was 14 years old. This sequence led to a beginning exploration of the patient's pathological mourning.

Session 5

The patient began by stating, "Nothing ever took root in my life." This statement heralded what was to be the adaptive context for this session: tragic loss resulting in a sense of impermanence and instability.

Sarah: Nothing took root ever in my life...parents, marriage, and now my son. After I went off with the teenage girls (in the

concentration camp), I had a sense of freedom like I'd never
had. There was my mother wanting to keep me with her, but
I wanted to get away from her, from her control over me.

Describes struggle with mother for autonomy as an adolescent.

Therapist: What was it like between the two of you?

*The therapist recognizes a decision point: either explore Sarah's leaving her
mother in the concentration camp or explore her prior relationship with her
mother. Rather than making the choice, the therapist asks an open-ended question, allowing Sarah to choose the most compelling direction.*

Sarah: My mother was a very strong woman. I remember that I
thought always that I was not deserving. My mother told me
that I was a child and I don't deserve it, whatever it was. It
was spelled out...I was only a child. I don't remember what
I did, but I was punished a lot...put in the corner...I know
I was ashamed because being punished proved I wasn't good.
I tried to be good.

*Chooses to talk about earlier experiences with mother in which her self-esteem
was diminished.*

Therapist: Your mother wanted you to be a certain way, well behaved, and when things went wrong you were punished, so
you thought you weren't good.

Clarifies.

The therapist continues to explore Sarah's early relationship with her
mother. It is helpful for the therapist to understand early relationship patterns and conflicts before undertaking an exploration of pathological
mourning.

Sarah: I did try, I was inconsolable when I was punished. I know
I peed in my underwear and tried to hide it. It made her very
angry when I was all wet and I tried to hide my clothes. I feel
humiliated, even now...to tell you this. It's going to sound
stupid, but I feel as a subject, judged and on the receiving
end, not in control.

Describes humiliating experience with mother and connects this with therapist.

Therapist: Judged by me and not in control, how is that?

Explores the subject of control, being judged, and self-esteem within the thera-peutic relationship.

Sarah: I'm uneasy talking this way.

Indicates that anxiety is increasing.

Therapist: So you're feeling anxious with me.

Clarifies anxiety.

Sarah: I think you'll write me off if I make a mistake.

Anxiety relates to fear of rejection and loss.

Therapist: And then what would happen?

Explores fantasy.

Sarah: It will be over between us.

Therapist: If you make a mistake with me?

Sarah: I made mistakes with my mother. Most things were forbid-den, but sometimes I defied her.

Links therapist with mother, indicating that she is able to readily use the ther-apeutic relationship in an adaptive manner.

Therapist: Do you recall a time when you defied your mother?

Sarah: *(Pause)*...I stole some fruit...maybe I was 7. Our neigh-bor had a fruit tree and the branch leaned over, almost on our property. My mother told me never to touch the neigh-bor's apples, but one day I picked some and later the neigh-bor approached me and asked if I took the fruit from her tree. I told her...that it was my mother who took the apples. When my mother found out, she cried and said, now the po-lice would come for her. Then I was scared about what would happen, but that time my mother didn't punish me.

Defies mother's prohibition.

Therapist: Hmm.

This type of utterance commonly used in psychotherapy invites patient to con-tinue.

Sarah: My mother was probably frightened for me that time...she may have been trying to keep me in line. Most things in my childhood were not for Jewish people...certain food and other things....Once in a while I used to think maybe I was at the top of the heap and had a favored position over my sisters (3 and 7 years the patient's junior). I remember at those times, my mother agreed with the things I said and I felt so good then. But I couldn't really believe I was favored.

Shifts emphasis to mother protecting her and thinking she may have been favored.

Therapist: Why was that?

Sarah: I had the idea that I wasn't a prize, like the others. My mother wanted a beautiful, popular daughter and I was un- gainly, even clumsy and unattractive. I had to get things in an underhanded way while my sisters were freely given to. I thought I was adopted, not really their daughter.

Shift back to negative view of self with the thought that she could be someone else's daughter. Sarah's automatic thought is "I am unattractive and have to get things in an underhanded way."

Therapist: So there were two contradictory thoughts. One was that occasionally you were at the top of the heap, and the other, more prevalent one was that you were a disappoint- ment to your mother. That must have been confusing.

Clarifies ambivalent thinking.

Sarah: *(Tearfully)* My mother was beautiful. My father thought she was a prize. When my father was away, she wanted me to sleep with her in her bed. When I was older she confided in me and I helped her with the family business. She said I had good business sense.

Describes closeness with mother.

Therapist: You and your mother were very close at times. Two women sharing something together.

Clarifies.

Sarah: Yes. But then my mother would send me out of the bed when my father returned, and it made me very angry. *(Sadly)* I didn't really understand what I'd done to deserve it.

Sarah's longing to remain with her mother is interfered with by the return of her father, and she believes that her mother preferred father.

> Therapist: How did you feel at those times? You said angry; anything else?

Explores feelings.

> Sarah: I learned to cut off from her. If she went one way I would go the other. I wanted to spite her...but...I really wanted to be with her *(sobbing)*.

Describes yearning for mother along with defensive oppositional behavior based on mother's rejection.

In this session, the patient was able to begin talking about her positive and negative feelings toward her mother. Sarah's underlying wish was to be close to and loved by her mother. When rejected, she became angry and oppositional, cutting her mother off. As a result of this, she developed dysfunctional thoughts of herself as an unattractive, adopted child, less favored than her siblings.

By the end of the session, the patient expresses her longings for her mother. The therapist's interventions were primarily clarifications and questions to further the process of exploration. The therapist was attentive to the therapeutic relationship, thereby maintaining a positive alliance.

Session 6

> Sarah: The last thing my mother asked me to do, before we went to the concentration camp, was to go to the cemetery to say goodbye to my grandfather. She had no time. She was getting ready to go. She had to pack and take care of my sisters. But I didn't go. I guess I didn't want to say goodbye and I didn't want to obey my mother.

Continues theme from previous session.

> Therapist: Earlier you told me that you chose to go with the older girls at the concentration camp and not remain with your mother.

> Sarah: I wanted freedom, to get away from her watchful eye. She died, my grandmother and sisters. I was the only one remaining alive. Even my father was killed later.

> Therapist: It was tragic....Were you able to say goodbye to
> them?

Now the therapist begins to explore the patient's devastating losses, beginning with that of her mother. It is crucial to explore significant losses in patient's lives, particularly if they result in pathological grief. Pathological mourning is generally the result of unresolved ambivalent feelings toward the lost person. In all psychotherapy, but particularly in brief psychotherapy, it is essential to explore unresolved grief early in treatment. Pathological grief can act as a barrier to the working through and resolution of other conflicts. Sarah had conflicts with her husband, her children, her supervisor at work, and the therapist that were related to her ambivalent relationship with and subsequent loss of her mother.

> Sarah: I left...never said goodbye to my mother. We just shook
> hands.

> Therapist: How did it actually happen?

Asks for specifics.

> Sarah: My mother wanted me to go with her. My grandmother
> and sisters were on one side with my mother. That's where
> most of the people were sent. I wanted to go with the big
> girls. I wanted to get away from my mother. She was always
> critical of me. I felt resentful of her. I was an awkward child.
> My grandmother liked me better than my mother did.

The therapist continues to explore many of the negative experiences with her mother and the resulting anger, frustration and humiliation. Following the exploration of the negative experiences and feelings, the therapist began to examine the patient's love and longing for her mother.

> Therapist: We've been talking about some of your negative feelings toward your mother, but we know you also had longings to be close to her.

> Sarah: My grandmother could have taken care of my sisters. My
> mother could have come with me.

Describes wish for mother to have gone with her and survived.

> Therapist: So you have the wish to be close to her, thinking that
> she should have chosen you.

Clarifies wish for mother.

Sarah: *(Tearfully)* But she didn't. They killed her and I never saw her again. I can't imagine what it was like. They had to get all undressed... naked. She hated for anyone to see her body. She should have come with me. We could have been together *(sobbing)*.

Generally, working through and resolving pathological mourning will take several sessions. The therapist needs to explore, in great detail, the events leading up to the loss of the person, the loss itself and the aftermath, including the funeral and burial when possible. The patient should be encouraged to express wishes and feelings toward the lost person. This enables individuals to go through the mourning process, which they could not do at the time of the loss. We can now understand why Sarah impulsively left her job when she was not selected for promotion by her boss. Her disappointment with her mother for favoring her father and her sisters appears to be linked to her behavior with her boss. Once the working through of pathological mourning is completed, other conflictual elements can be explored in a productive manner. If pathological mourning is not dealt with first, other conflicts are much more difficult to work with.

Case 4: Expressive Psychotherapy—
The Man Who Never Said Goodbye

Mark is a 42-year-old married man with two young daughters who works for a major corporation in a middle-management position. His three most troubling problems were 1) episodes of rage, at times with strangers; 2) inability to pursue career goals, which is related to interpersonal passivity; and 3) conflictual problems in his marriage.

In general, the patient was a passive man who seemed to agreeably accede to the wishes of others. Prior to entering treatment, Mark began to have angry, unpredictable outbursts when frustrated by others. His last outburst resulted in an arrest for disorderly conduct, which impelled him to seek treatment.

There were many losses in his early life. When Mark was 3 years old, his father died of cancer after a brief illness. Then his mother, who began to drink heavily after his father's death, died in a car accident 18 months later. After that, the patient went to live with an aunt and uncle, who raised him. As a young adult, Mark was in psychotherapy for several years.

Session 1

In the first session, Mark described the three major complaints outlined above. After an initial survey, the therapist began by exploring the patient's angry outbursts.

> Therapist: Let's examine your angry outbursts in more detail. Can you give me an example of a recent occurrence?

Therapist asks for a concrete example.

> Mark: Well let's see...I was downtown, driving around, looking for a parking spot. I saw a guy get into his car so I pulled up and waited in front of him. As he pulled out, someone came from behind and just pulled into the spot. I started screaming at this guy.

Patient is able to give a clear example, indicating that he is well motivated and not highly resistant.

> Therapist: You were furious with him.

Underlines anger.

> Mark: Yes, what was he trying to do?

> Therapist: How did you experience being angry with him?

Asks for the patient's experience of the affect. In short-term dynamic psychotherapy, an in-depth exploration of affect with a patient on the right side of the continuum can lead to a breakthrough of underlying unconscious material, which will further the therapeutic alliance and shorten the treatment.

> Mark: I got so angry I blocked his car with mine. I kept screaming at him.

Avoids expressing inner experience.

> Therapist: Before we get to what you did, let's try to understand what you were experiencing within yourself. How did you experience your anger toward him inside yourself?

Continues to focus on Mark's inner experience.

> Mark: I threatened to kill him. I shoved him by the shoulders, but then he moved away.

Defensively avoids inner experience.

> Therapist: Do you notice that you shifted, describing how you behaved, rather than what you felt within yourself.

The therapist is working within the triangle of conflict and attempting to get a clear description of the patient's feeling toward this stranger. However, the patient bypasses his inner experience of anger by immediately describing his behavioral response. This indicates that the patient may have a tendency to act out his feelings rather than attend to his inner experience. The therapeutic task for this patient is to fully experience his feeling, both emotionally and cognitively, so that he can cope with frustration more adaptively.

> Therapist: We'll get to what you did later. For now, let's try to see how you experience the anger within yourself.

Continues to confront patient.

> Mark: I felt like I was burning up inside. I was in a rage.

Able to describe inner experience.

> Therapist: So there was an inner feeling of rage, a burning up within yourself. What else did you experience physically?

Clarifies and asks Mark to elaborate further.

> Mark: I felt a tightness in my chest, my face was burning up (clenches fist).

Describes physiological response (burning up) and displays a motoric reaction (clenched fist).

> Therapist: And as you were experiencing these feelings, you shoved him. Did you want to hurt him?

Shifts from exploration of anger to Mark's aggressive wish or fantasy, completing the three components of a fully experienced feeling. The three elements making up the inner experience of affect are 1) physiological arousal; 2) motoric manifestation of activation, such as raised voice and body movement; and 3) cognitive acknowledgment of inner urges and fantasy (Laikin et al. 1991).

> Mark: I felt like killing him and I threatened him, but I would never do that. It's wrong (becomes visibly anxious).

> Therapist: So having these thoughts and feelings of wanting to kill him are frightening and cause you anxiety.

Links anxiety to aggressive wish. The patient's expression of anger and wish to kill led to significant anxiety. When the patient becomes anxious, the therapist, using the triangle of conflict, generally should stop exploring the affect of anger and shift to an exploration of anxiety. Such a shift should help to decrease the level of anxiety so that further investigation of the patient's anger and fantasy can continue.

Therapist: Tell me about the anxiety; how do you experience it?

Mark: I feel a pounding, my heart is pounding. It really scares me to think I could feel like killing him.

Therapist: There is a big difference between feeling or thinking about killing him and doing it. It's very important to see the difference between the thought of killing and the actual act of killing. You had the thought accompanied by strong feelings.

Separates feelings and wishes from action. Explanations of this kind constitute a cognitive restructuring process and are helpful to patients who blur the distinction between thoughts or feelings and actions.

Mark: Yes, but it's hard to talk about.

Therapist: It's important for us to fully explore your fantasy about killing him so we can understand your feelings of rage.

Asks patient to continue in a collaborative manner.

Mark: I wanted to hurt him, punch him, make him suffer.

Expresses his wish.

Therapist: So you were furious and had a strong wish to hurt him. What did you do in actuality?

Clarifies patient's affect and wish and then asks for actual behavior.

Mark explained that he withdrew from the confrontation and drove away, but felt weak and defeated by the incident. The therapist commented that one of Mark's major complaints was his passivity. The patient agreed, and told the therapist that this was most problematic at work. The therapist asked for an example.

Mark: My supervisor at work was critical.

Therapist: His name is?

It is always helpful to obtain first names of important people in the patient's life. Use of such people's first names makes the therapy come alive and enables patients to be more in touch with their inner lives.

> Mark: Elliot. He was critical and nasty, and then I started to get angry at him.

> Therapist: How did you experience the anger toward Elliot?

Asks for inner experience of affect.

> Mark: That son of a bitch, he doesn't know what he's doing, but I can't tell him anything. I have to keep my mouth shut.

Expresses some anger, but indicates that he became passive in this situation.

> Therapist: You have powerful feelings toward him but you hold back and make yourself passive. Then you erupt with other people like the man who took the parking space. It's either one extreme or the other.

Points out his extremes in behavior.

> Mark: It's hard for me; I sort of lose myself, I don't remember.

> Therapist: Now you have become vague with me in relation to your feelings. When you have powerful feelings, you have an array of defenses to deal with these feelings, like vagueness, passivity, avoidance, and not remembering.

Summarizes the patient's use of a number of defenses to ward off his intolerable feelings. By naming these defenses—vagueness, passivity, avoidance, and forgetting—the therapist acquaints the patient with his characteristic defensive style. The therapist is helping the patient to understand the triangle of conflict.

> Mark: I get afraid I'll lose control completely, like in the parking incident. If I have an impulse to kill someone, I become terrified.

Continues to express fear of acting on his impulses.

> Therapist: Let's look at that fear and terror; what is that like for you?

> Mark: It's complete fear. I'm powerless. I can't get what I want. I can't get anything. He's powerful and menacing. I look to be cared for.

Indicates that his fear leads to feelings of powerlessness and a wish to be cared for.

> Therapist: How does that apply here with me—do you feel the same way toward me?

The therapist senses that the patient may be having a similar reaction within the therapeutic relationship.

> Mark: You're confronting me about things I don't want to get to.

> Therapist: If I hang back, what will happen to our work together?

The therapist has uncovered the patient's fear of his aggression coupled with his wish to be cared for. The therapist appeals to the patient's observing ego to further the therapeutic alliance.

The remainder of this initial session was devoted to an exploration of the patient's work, marital history, and past history. The goals of treatment were discussed and agreed upon.

> Therapist: As we've seen today, which you said earlier, you have three major problems. First, you have a problem controlling your anger: either you erupt without thinking or you behave in a passive or unassertive manner, which extends to the second problem area of work and the third area, with your wife. You've also had terrible losses early in your life. How would you feel about working on these problems the way we have today?

> Mark: I would like that. I want to do better for myself and my family.

The therapist's review of Mark's major problem areas sets the stage for their agreement on the goals of therapy (see Treatment Plan below for further discussion of goals).

Case Formulation

Structural Approach

The major structural impairment is in the area of impulse control. The patient's angry outbursts have led to major problems culminating in his recent arrest. At other times he is overly controlled, which results in extreme passivity. Mark's reality testing is intact, but his judgment can be impaired when he is frustrated. The patient has powerful affects of anger and sadness. His major defenses are passivity, avoidance, forgetting, and vagueness.

In the area of object relations, the patient has achieved object constancy and has triadic relationships. In times of stress, he regresses, and his relationships, which are generally give-and-take, become based more on need satisfaction. Mark's sense of self is that he is powerless and weak, which results in an absence of self-esteem and confidence.

Genetic Approach

The central traumas in the patient's life were the loss of his father at age 3 and his mother 18 months later. These losses occurred during the Oedipal period, which may have heightened Mark's sense of responsibility for their deaths. After the loss of his parents, Mark went to live with his aunt and uncle, who took care of him until age 10, when his aunt died and his uncle became ill. Again he sustained significant losses and was unable to mourn. Mark then went to live with his married brother, who was 17 years his senior. He had a conflictual relationship with his brother and sister-in-law, who he felt were unable to satisfy his needs.

Dynamic Approach

Mark has a number of wishes and needs. The central conflict involves the wish (W) to be loved and cared for, as expressed to the therapist in the evaluation. He defends against this wish by becoming passive or avoidant, but when others disappoint him (R_O) for not understanding his needs, he becomes furious at them and/or self-sabotaging or passive (R_S).

As a child, Mark sustained numerous losses. His difficulty in expressing his needs and asserting himself in part derives from these early losses. Close relationships are difficult for him, because he has a continuing fear of losing anyone he gets close to. At the same time, Mark is afraid to be active and assertive with others, fearing that his aggression is somehow connected to the losses in his life.

Cognitive-Behavioral Approach

The problem list consists of poor judgment when frustrated and inappropriate anger, passivity, inability to pursue career goals, and marital conflicts. Mark's automatic thoughts are "If I get angry, I'll lose control," "If I stand up for myself, I'll lose important people in my life," and "Others are more powerful than I am." His core belief is that he can't get what he wants from others because he is weak and powerless. The origins of this belief are the loss of his parents and other caretakers at an early age. Mark's arrest following the altercation led him to pursue treatment. The working hypothesis is that is that the patient's inappropriate anger and passivity are based on his core belief that he is powerless and unable to satisfy his needs, which was activated by a situation in which he was frustrated and unable to get what he needed. Possible obstacles to treatment are the time limit, in the sense that Mark may have difficulty acknowledging his progress and giving up the therapist and he may also experience the time limit as frustrating and withholding, which may interfere with the therapeutic relationship.

Diagnostic Evaluation

Axis I	None
Axis II	Personality disorder NOS with obsessional, dependent, and passive-aggressive features
Axis III	None
Axis IV	Work-related stress
Axis V	GAF = 74

Treatment Plan

Trial therapy with Mark indicates that he is able to work in an expressive mode, which places him on the right side of the continuum. His response to interventions addressing his defensive behavior and maladaptive patterns indicates an ability to benefit from a highly exploratory approach. He was able to express his feelings in a direct manner and elaborated on some of his fantasies, indicating a positive therapeutic alliance. The immediate treatment goal will be to understand Mark's current behavioral polarities of either acting out in an aggressive and inappropriate manner or resorting to passive or helpless defensive stances. Both positive and negative affects, particularly anger, need to be mobilized, fully experienced, and then cognitively integrated. Cognitive integration and restructuring is critical to enable Mark to gain mastery over his impulses while learning to assert himself in an adaptive manner. The cognitive and emotional task is for Mark to experience his anger and respond in ways that are appropriately assertive (ultimate goal). This issue should be worked through with important figures in his current and past life, and in the transference. During the midphase of treatment, another ultimate goal will be working through the loss of his parents and other significant persons early in his life. In the termination phase, the loss of the therapist will provide an opportunity for the patient to experience loss without the finality of death.

Session 4

> Mark: I was uncomfortable with the last session. You had an agenda that you imposed on me. You wanted to find out about my past treatment...I wanted to talk about what was on my mind. Just like when I was a kid...nobody let me express what I wanted. It's also related to the time limit on therapy—knowing this, I can't settle in, I have to keep the end in mind. I have to protect myself.

Criticizes therapist for not allowing him to express himself (an imposition that reminds him of his past experiences), then raises the issue of brief therapy. Although the patient's criticism represents a rupture in the therapeutic alliance, it also reflects a departure from Mark's previous behavior of avoiding conflict. Here he is appropriately assertive with the therapist.

> Therapist: These are important issues. Let's look more carefully at what you experience. We know it's connected to the past, but let's look at your feelings here with me.

Focuses on patient-therapist relationship.

> Mark: I wanted to talk about my immediate feelings of stress at work.

Avoids his feelings toward therapist.

> Therapist: So this was on your mind when I was asking about your previous therapy. How did you feel toward me at that time?

Holds patient to the patient-therapist relationship and patient's inner feelings.

> Mark: Well, you were asking me questions; I was getting irritated.

Expresses feeling.

> Therapist: So you were angry with me. How did you experience the anger toward me?

Restates that patient was angry and asks for inner experience.

Mark: I was annoyed. Issues about my parents kept coming up, so that part was good, but I was annoyed by your agenda.

Therapist: So you were annoyed with me about my agenda. What did you do with that annoyance or anger?

Recognizes that Mark was angry during the last session but withheld his anger.

Mark: I pushed it down, but there's so much on my mind. I want to get everything on the table.

Therapist: You're feeling that with me now, some annoyance?

Elicits Mark's feeling toward therapist at present time.

Mark: Yes.

Therapist: You felt that with me last time, but you held back. Let's try to understand that.

Explores patient's defensiveness.

Mark: When I left, I realized something was bothering me.

Partially avoids.

Therapist: So something was there on your mind, but you couldn't come out with it.

Continues confronting.

Mark: Yes, but what you were asking was important.

Defensive rationalization.

Therapist: I understand that you felt that my questions were important, but let's try to focus in on the other side. What was holding you back?

Maintains focus.

Mark: I would have been violating what you were doing. I went along with you.

Passive stance.

Therapist: So what do you think about this? We know this is an issue in your life. You go along and later explode.

Interprets patient's passivity as a defense against anger.

Mark: This is an issue in my life. It's in my marriage...in my job. There's lots of talk about technicalities at work. I have emotions, strong ones, but what can I do with emotions at work? You were dealing with facts, too. I wanted to talk about my emotions.

Recognizes that passivity is pervasive in his life.

Therapist: What would have happened if you brought this up last time, your annoyance and anger with me? What would have happened between us?

Focuses on Mark's anger and asks for a fantasy.

Mark: I'm trying to think...I guess my fear was you wouldn't be able to deal with my feelings. You'd disappoint me like my brother. You would have avoided the issue and defended yourself. You wouldn't deal with my feelings...my anger toward you. Yet I also know you probably could have.

Presents a two-sided obsessional description of how therapist might respond.

Therapist: So part of you realizes that I would have listened and been able to hear your feelings. Yet you couldn't come to grips with that.

Points out that Mark realizes the difference between his expectation of others and his expectation of the therapist (transference).

Mark: Yes *(begins to cry)*. Like Sue, my wife. She can understand my feelings. She listens to me. She sees my shortcomings, but she still loves me *(more tears)*.

Expresses strong feelings and connects them to his wife.

Therapist: So she loves you, listens, and understands. And the tears?

Clarification and exploration of affect.

Mark: This makes her a wonderful mother to our children. She's like the mother I never had.

Expresses longing for an understanding mother.

> Therapist: So the tears relate to this...strong positive feelings for Sue.

> Mark: I feel touched. She wasn't in my life early on, but she can understand what happened to me. I always wanted people to know what happened to me...to understand. On the other hand, I can't be direct with her...like we're talking here, the way I'm talking with you.

Expresses positive regard for therapist.

> Therapist: And if you were direct with her, what would happen?

Focuses on avoidance with wife.

> Mark: There would be a lot of anger expressed back and forth. She would work through the anger, but I can't. I avoid it with her.

Recognizes his defensive behavior.

> Therapist: So you avoid it with Sue, and we saw you avoided your feelings with me and being direct with me.

Transference interpretation linking avoidance of feeling with wife and therapist.

> Mark: In retrospect, I could have done it with you; with her it's more difficult. There's more conflict, but she's willing to work on it, to try to solve it.

> Therapist: Your tendency is to always keep your feeling back and hide it, you avoid. Last week you were afraid that I would ignore you, not pay attention to you, or that I might react negatively, even retaliate.

Holds patient to his feelings toward therapist in order to explore and repair the misalliance.

> Mark: How could you ask such matter-of-fact questions? I opened up to you, and last week...the questions, I got angry and started to see you negatively. I didn't stop you, but I got angry. I'm filled with memories and tears. Also, what you were asking me about made me feel uncomfortable. They are important issues, so maybe I was trying to avoid those things.

Again expresses anger toward therapist, then obsessionally shifts to the importance of therapist's questions.

> Therapist: So we've come full circle. Now you're starting to blame yourself and question yourself.

> Mark: Yes, things are complex. I'm taking back my anger, but I also realize that what you were bringing up was important.

> Therapist: Okay, both things can be true, but your initial feeling is still your feeling. Now you're making it less important, pushing it back under the table.

Points out defensive avoidance.

> Mark: I like to see the whole picture.

Rationalizes.

> Therapist: But your feeling is still your feeling…by making it more complicated, you obliterate your feeling and what we did together. You push things down.

Continues to hold patient to the issue at hand.

> Mark: I should have said to you, I don't want to talk about my prior treatment. I have other things on my mind and also why I didn't want to talk about those things.

The patient takes a stand with the therapist and is able to assert himself in an effective manner. This is one of many experiences in which the patient is able to be direct with the therapist and express negative feeling. Since there is no retaliation, Mark learns that he can express his feelings directly. This provides the patient with a "corrective emotional experience" (Alexander and French 1946; see Chapters 1 and 5). In the remainder of this session, the patient spoke about his difficulties in being direct with his wife and began to understand that he fears her anger and being abandoned by her.

Conclusions

In this chapter we have presented the beginning phase of treatment of four patients at different points on the psychological structure/psychotherapy continuum. The major tasks of the initial phase of treatment are as follows:

1) establish a positive therapeutic relationship with the patient, 2) complete a thorough assessment and diagnostic formulation to determine the patients' place on the continuum, 3) set goals, and 4) apply an integrative approach, using appropriate interventions.

The beginning phase of therapy involves a learning process for both patient and therapist. Patients become acquainted with the therapeutic process, which may be explicitly or implicitly educative, and learn about the nature of their problems and the therapist's style and approach. Likewise, therapists come to know about their patients, arrive at a formulation of their problems, and establish rapport with them.

CHAPTER

8

Midphase of Treatment

In the midphase of an integrated treatment, the emphasis is on a working-through, problem-solving, and/or building process. There is less uncovering or learning about the patient and more working through, problem resolution, and cognitive restructuring and/or structure building. Patients continue to learn about themselves and to apply what they have learned to their problematic ways of behaving and thinking. In an integrated treatment approach, the work of the midphase depends on where the individual is on the psychopathology–psychological structure continuum. Patients on the left side of the continuum—those with more psychopathology—will do best with a structure-building approach, whereas those on the right side of the continuum—those with less psychopathology—will benefit most from a working-through process.

In expressive psychotherapy, the midphase emphasis is on the working-through process. Greenson (1967, p. 42) described *working through* as follows:

Working through refers to a complex set of procedures and processes which occur after an insight has been given....It refers in the main to the repetitive, progressive and elaborate explorations of the resistances which prevent an insight from leading to change.... A variety of circular processes are set in motion by working through in which insight, memory and behavior change influence each other.

In brief dynamic psychotherapy, the circular process must be rapidly mobilized and accompanied by appropriate affect so that working through does not become an intellectual exercise. To accomplish this, the therapist must be clear about the central issues and the core conflict of the patient. The components of working through—memory, affect, insight, and behavior change—interact with one another in the manner of a feedback loop or circular process and can be blocked by patient resistance. Resistance must constantly be confronted, clarified, and interpreted so that working through can proceed. Working through must occur in many areas of the patient's life. For example, a 38-year-old man repeatedly finds himself in conflict with authority figures. This conflict must be worked through with his boss, co-workers, parents, and the therapist so that it can be resolved.

In supportive psychotherapy, conflict generally plays a less important or a secondary role. Structural deficits are primary, so that a more reparative approach is needed. The primary goals of supportive psychotherapy are building self-esteem, improving psychological (ego) functioning, and promoting adaptation. By midphase the therapist and patient should have identified what needs to be done in these areas. The "working through" in supportive psychotherapy as well as cognitive-behavioral therapy involves learning new ways of thinking and behaving leading to enhanced self-esteem and so is more of a building process. Enhanced self-esteem enables the patient to continue the process of learning and behaving in a more productive manner. This cycle, based on repetitive learning in the context of a good therapeutic relationship, constitutes the building process of supportive psychotherapy.

For patients closer to the middle of the continuum, a combined approach of working through and a building process is needed. Balance between these two approaches will depend on the therapist's structural assessment of the patient. As described earlier, patients with more serious pathology will require more support, whereas patients with fewer deficits will benefit from an approach that uses a greater number of expressive techniques. In the midphase of treatment, the more expressive the therapy, the greater the use of working through. Supportive psychotherapy will rely more on a building process during the midphase.

Case 1: Supportive Psychotherapy— The Woman Who Lived on the Edge

By the fourth week of treatment, Lucy's mood had noticeably improved. Her depression lifted, sleep and appetite disturbance diminished, and she began to care for her baby. Anxiety and panic symptoms also diminished, and her suicidal thoughts disappeared. As stated earlier, the goal of supportive psychotherapy is to improve psychological (ego) functioning, adaptation, and self-esteem. The patient's ability to care for her daughters and herself provided evidence of improved psychological and adaptive functioning.

Session 7

Lucy appeared to be downhearted, kept her outer jacket on, and propped her head up on her hands. She was silent.

> Therapist: How is it going?

The therapist is aware that the patient is concerned about something and looks downhearted, but asks a general question. It might have been better to immediately focus on the patient's affect.

> Lucy: My brother is going back to Florida tomorrow. He has to get back to his nursing job; they need him at the hospital.

The patient responds directly and concretely to the therapist's general question.

> Therapist: What are your thoughts about Isaac's *(her brother)* leaving?

> Lucy: I knew he would only be here for 2 weeks, but I want him to stay. He helps with Brenda and the baby.

> Therapist What will it be like tomorrow when he leaves and you're alone with Brenda and Crystal *(baby)*?

Asks patient to anticipate.

> Lucy: *(Tearful)* I want to go with him....

> Therapist: And...?

> Lucy: I know I can't...he'll be working, and he has to see his children, too. But I.... *(Patient begins to weep.)*

Recognizes her conflict; her wish to be with her brother, and her realization that she cannot go with him.

Therapist: What thoughts are bringing the tears?

Asks for thoughts to help patient develop a cognitive framework and promote intellectualization and understanding.

Lucy: I'm helpless again, just like when Brenda was a baby. Only now I have two children.

Regresses to a helpless state, but is able to make a connection to the past.

Therapist: So are the tears about thinking you're inadequate to care for yourself and your daughters?

Linking affect with thoughts and clarifying.

Lucy: I guess so...yes.

Therapist: It's your thought, but is it true?

Challenges automatic thinking.

Lucy: I wouldn't leave her the way I left Brenda.

Indicates greater responsibility for her infant.

Therapist: Well, back then you were only 22 years old, in a strange city with no friends, and you didn't think you could survive the nights alone...I mean, with Carl away. Now you're more mature and responsible.

Provides a rationalization for past behavior and praises her current thinking.

Lucy: Well, yeah...but Carl (*husband*) still goes away...and John (*boyfriend*)...it's over with him. He doesn't return my calls...he doesn't want anything to do with me.

Therapist: With all these men leaving, Isaac, John, and Carl, you're having a rough time. Although they are all leaving in one way or another, it would be helpful to examine your thoughts about each one separately, since they are leaving for different reasons. Does that make sense?

*Clarifies losses in an empathic manner. An attempt is made to divide a compli-
cated problem into smaller parts to elicit dysfunctional thinking and then seek
collaboration in problem solving and changing automatic thinking.*

> Lucy: Yeah, Isaac has to go back to his work and daughters;
> I guess he cares about them.

*Responds to therapist and focuses on her brother, but hints that he may not care
about her.*

> Therapist: Yes, he must care about them, but he also cares about
> you. Didn't he choose to take time from work and leave his
> daughters to help you?

Continues to work on challenging negative thinking and enhancing self-esteem.

> Lucy: Yeah, I guess I'm important to him, but not as important as
> his daughters or work.

> Therapist: We've talked about these automatic thoughts before;
> you are assuming that you're not worth much because Isaac
> is going back to his job and family. Your automatic thought is
> "Isaac loves his family more than me, therefore I am no good."

States automatic thought linking it to self-esteem.

> Lucy: Yes, you're right, it doesn't make sense, but that's how I see
> it. That's how I am.

Resists and holds fast to her automatic thought.

> Therapist: Yes, that's your usual way of thinking and it's hard to
> change, but this kind of thinking, reaching negative conclu-
> sions, ends up making you feel like you're not worth any-
> thing much.

*Acknowledges difficulty changing and continues to work on negative thinking
and self-esteem.*

Lucy exhibits dysfunctional thinking, leading to problems in self-esteem.
In the midphase of therapy, working on dysfunctional thinking constitutes
one of the major approaches for patients with poor structure and depressive
symptoms. The therapist repeatedly identifies and explores automatic thoughts
and other forms of dysfunctional thinking. This needs to be undertaken with
important persons in the patient's life in different types of situations.

Session 10

> Lucy: I couldn't get a baby-sitter, so I brought the baby with me...is it okay?

Seeks approval from the therapist.

> Therapist: It's fine. Bringing Crystal here is a good idea. It took care of the baby-sitter problem and gave me a chance to meet her. She's so alert, and you have her dressed so nicely!

Praises problem-solving ability and is admiring of how Lucy is caring for Crystal.

> Lucy: Since I've been feeling better, I can really pay attention to her. I can take care of her and dress her up. I even get up with her at night...Brenda doesn't have to do it anymore.

> Therapist: That's terrific. Does that make you feel better about yourself?

Acknowledges adaptive functioning and continues to praise.

> Lucy: Yes, but I still don't feel good about John. John doesn't want anything to do with me. I don't call him anymore, but I miss him.

Shifts to another problem area.

> Therapist: What do you miss about him?

Therapist might have pointed out Lucy's change of subject, but instead followed the patient's lead.

> Lucy: I had a lot of fun with him. He took me out, we did things together, he gave me attention and took care of me. One time he let the water into the tub for my bath.

> Therapist: So these are the things that make you miss him, he gave you attention. How about the other part of your relationship with him?

Refocuses on John's negative attributes.

> Lucy: What do you mean?

> Therapist: You are talking about all your positive thoughts and memories, but wasn't he also brutal toward you?

Addresses Lucy's defensive forgetting.

> Lucy: You mean, when he put the pillow over my face and beat me when I didn't buy him sunglasses.

> Therapist: That's one time...he could have killed you...don't you think?

> Lucy: Um...I know, but I end up feeling sorry for him, even though I ended up all bruised. He always wanted to do everything his way. And blaming me for his messed-up life.

Allows that he treated her badly, but indicates that she felt sorry for him.

> Therapist: So when you are missing John, it's the attention he gave you that you think about. You forget all the horrible things he did and said to you.

Clarifies.

> Lucy: I don't know why I do that.

> Therapist: I don't know if you will agree, but I think your wish for closeness and a caring relationship distorts the way you see John. You eliminate all the awful things he did to you from your thinking.

Continues to address dysfunctional thinking.

Toward the end of this session, the therapist suggested that Lucy keep a record of her negative thoughts so that automatic thoughts could be more readily identified by the patient and then reviewed in therapy sessions. This session began with Lucy bringing her infant daughter into the office. In supportive psychotherapy, this not only is permissible but also can be helpful. In contrast, expressive psychotherapy should provide less direct gratification of the patient. When Lucy came to the session with her daughter, a number of adaptive changes could be seen. She was motivated to attend the session and able to problem-solve and to take care of her daughter. The therapist praised Lucy's adaptive behavior with a view toward enhancing her self-esteem.

During this session, Lucy talked about missing her boyfriend, John, who was an abusive man. The therapist identified Lucy's dysfunctional thinking by pointing out her selective way of thinking and remembering. The therapist is aware of the patient's past history of abuse and neglect at the hands of her mother, father, and stepmother. These experiences are connected to her longing for John, regardless of his behavior toward her. In brief supportive psychotherapy, these links to the past are generally not made. Instead, the therapist concentrates on problems in the patient's current life.

Session 12

In the beginning of this session, the therapist focuses on psychopharmacological issues as a result of Lucy's question about how long she will need to remain on the antidepressant medication.

> Lucy: You know…I'm feeling much better…not down anymore.

> Therapist: Yes, you are doing a lot better.

Acknowledges progress.

> Lucy: I don't like taking medication. Since I'm feeling better I'm thinking about going back to work and I want to stop the medicine.

> Therapist: Well, let's see. You began the medication about 3 months ago and you've made a lot of progress. I know you would rather not take anything, and many people feel the same way but do better by staying on the medication. Is there anything else going on, are you having side effects from the medication?

Asks Lucy about side effects of the medication. A common reason for a patient to stop medication is uncomfortable side effects.

> Lucy: No, I'm not having any problems with it, except I don't want to be on it forever.

> Therapist: Yes, I know what you mean, but if you stop the medication, the chances of relapsing—getting depressed or having panic attacks again—are much more likely. Studies indicate that the relapse rate for depression is in the neighborhood of 90%, so if you go off the medication, there's a good chance that you'll get sick again.

> Lucy: Dr. Green (*family practitioner*) says the same thing. He told me to continue the medicine, but it makes me think that I'm still sick.

> Therapist: Well, maybe if you start to think about it differently it will help. You're thinking, "If I take the antidepressant, it means I'm sick," when actually it is the medication that helps keep you well! The kind of depression you've struggled with all your life is a medical condition. You know, if you had diabetes or heart disease, you would probably need to be on medication for the rest of your life to keep you well, and you would have to periodically consult with a physician about your condition. Well, it's similar with depression.

Many patients who take psychoactive medication struggle with the idea that they need to remain on medication for an extended period of time or even for the rest of their lives. Recent research findings suggest that patients with recurrent major depression do better remaining on antidepressant medication. The risk of relapse after a third episode of major depression is approximately 90% for an unmedicated patient, and subsequent episodes often occur sooner, are of longer duration, and are more severe and less responsive to treatment (Angst 1999; Angst et al. 1973; Keller et al. 1992; Lavori et al. 1994). During the initial sessions, Lucy was given information about the medication and told she would need to be on the medication for a long time. It is not unusual for patients who begin to feel less depressed to think about stopping—or in fact to stop—the medication. The therapist needs to be prepared for this problem by using the most recent research findings to educate the patient about medication.

Case 2: Supportive-Expressive Psychotherapy— The Woman Who Thought She Was a Murderer

The initial phase of treatment for Christine focused on providing stability through the use of supportive measures to reduce anxiety, to alleviate her guilt about Tom's death, and to address cognitive distortions. This focus helped her to return to work and to begin to socialize again. Although there was some exploration of the traumatic event during the initial phase, in-depth work on Christine's trauma began during the midphase of treatment and continued through the termination phase. The midphase for Christine was characterized by working through a number of traumatic dreams.

Session 5

Christine entered the therapist's office and appeared to be uncomfortable.

> Christine: I'm still having nightmares.

Therapist: Tell me about one of the nightmares.

Therapist asks for an example.

Christine: Last night I had one. A man stopped me when I was walking. He called me names. People stopped and stared. Then he shoved me up against a fence...hard. He slapped my bag out of my hands and started punching me. I tried to move away from him, but he wouldn't let me. It woke me up, I was so scared.

The patient presents a focused account of a recent frightening nightmare.

Therapist: Yes, that's pretty scary. Let's try to understand what it means.

Christine: Since I was shot, I've been having nightmares like this.

Connects nightmares with shooting.

Therapist: The shooting was so traumatic to you that it's with you most of the time, even when you're sleeping.

Makes supportive statements, helping the patient to continue focusing on the nightmare and the traumatic events that shattered her life and brought her into psychotherapy.

Therapist: Did you recognize the man in the dream?

Christine: I...think it was Tom's brother...Patrick. It looked like him. He hates me now, since Tom killed himself. He blames me and he's crazy, he uses drugs—they all do, the whole family. They all blame me. His mother told my friend Patty that if he'd had a different girlfriend, he'd be okay, you know, alive today.

Indicates that others are blaming her for Tom's death.

Therapist: They blame you, but that doesn't mean that they know what they're talking about. One of the problems we need to work on is that you blame yourself. Let's look at your journal to see what kind of thoughts you've been having.

Identifies dysfunctional thinking and asks about journal.

Christine: Well, this is what I wrote about Tom. I keep thinking I could have done things differently, I shouldn't have left him.

Identifies an automatic thought, "If I had stayed with Tom, he would be alive today."

> Therapist: How would it have been if you had remained with him?—because we know he physically brutalized you.

> Christine: I couldn't have, we had nothing, he was always yelling at me. We never did anything or went anyplace. He didn't seem to even care about me.

The therapist continued to confront Christine with the reality of her relationship with Tom in order to promote a realistic appraisal of Tom's treatment of her to cast doubts about her responsibility for his death. Realistically appraising her relationship with Tom will enable her to understand that her feelings of responsibility and guilt for his suicide are cognitive distortions. Her nightmares are multidetermined and demonstrate her attempt to work through the traumatic experience as well as her feelings of guilt.

> Therapist: Let's try to understand more about the nightmare.

> Christine: Patrick was hitting and pushing me.... I was so scared.

> Therapist: So you continue to get battered.

Notes that patient continues to punish herself.

> Christine: I still think so much about what happened. I can't get it out of my head.

> Therapist: It's still very much with you. It seems to me that we need to go into the details of the shootings, Tom shooting you, Tom's suicide, your surgery...all of it. I know it's hard for you, you became very distressed when we first talked about it, but now you're doing better. Do you feel able to talk some more about it now?

Proposes taking patient through the traumatic experience (exposure), but checks to see if she is willing to proceed.

> Christine: I think so. It's with me so much of the time anyway.

> Therapist: Let's go back to the actual shootings. Tell me what happened?

> Christine: I was walking home from work.... Tom drove up and stopped. He told me to get in the car. I didn't want to, but I didn't want to make a scene, so I got in.

Therapist: How did he appear? What did he look like?

Asks for details in order to paint a portrait of the event.

Christine: He was yelling...screaming. He looked crazy.

Therapist: How did you feel?

Christine: I was scared *(appears visibly anxious)*. He was calling me a whore.

Therapist: What else did he say?

Helps patient elaborate.

Christine: He said, "I know you have a boyfriend, you whore." I wanted to get out of the car, but he was holding my wrist so tight I thought my arm would break. Then he pulled out the gun.

Therapist: And you were feeling?

Christine: I was scared to death. I thought he was going to kill me. I didn't know what to do.

Therapist: And then what happened?

Christine: He shot me. I heard the gunshots.... He shot me twice in the stomach.

Therapist: And the pain?

Christine: It felt like my body exploded *(gestures, holding abdominal area)*. Somehow I managed to get out of the car...he must have let go of me.... I crawled onto the sidewalk...he shot me again.

Relives the traumatic event in the presence of a benign figure.

Therapist: My God! It must have been horrible.

Christine: I tried to call for help. I could hardly call out. I kept dragging myself to the front of a house.

Therapist: Then what?

Christine: A woman came out of the house, she saw me. I thought I was going to die. The next thing I knew I was waking up in the hospital. I had tubes coming out of me everywhere. My mother was crying.

Therapist: So Tom almost succeeded in killing you.

Christine: Yes, it's true.

Therapist: And in the dream, his brother continues hurting you. It just doesn't end. You go on suffering.

Links the actual event with Tom's brother in the nightmare in an empathic manner.

Christine: Yes, again and again. I can't get away from it.

Presents passive, helpless position.

Therapist: I can see that's true. In the dream, Patrick beats you up the way Tom did. You endure suffering in this dream and in real life as well.

Points out that patient continues to suffer.

Christine: I can't help it. I keep thinking I started it all by leaving him.

Returns to her automatic thought.

Therapist: Well you did leave him, but you did the reasonable thing by leaving a brutal and violent man. Your decision was sound.

Presents evidence to challenge Christine's automatic thought.

Christine: You're right...he was no good...I had nothing with him for years.

Allows that her decision might have been correct.

The session continued with further exploration of the shootings, Tom's suicide, and her feelings of guilt and responsibility for what happened.

Session 7

The patient, until now, has expressed little in the way of negative feelings toward Tom. In this session, these feelings began to emerge, but she was unable to fully express them because she still feared Tom and at times fantasized that he was still alive. Once she begins to accept the reality of his death, the mourning process can go forward and her true feelings toward him can emerge.

> Christine: I've been thinking something stupid...I don't know how to say it. Is he really dead? I was in the hospital when he was buried. I keep thinking he'll turn up.

Denies Tom's death.

> Therapist: What's stupid about that? Remember we talked about your habit of devaluing what you think and devaluing yourself as a person.

Supports patient's self-esteem.

> Christine: I know you're right...I do that...but I'm still afraid of him.

> Therapist: Are you afraid of your thoughts or feelings about him?

Recognizes that the patient has negative thoughts or feelings toward Tom.

> Christine: I don't know, I don't like how I feel.

Vague response, avoiding true feelings.

> Therapist: It's hard to come out with what you really feel about Tom.

Empathic confrontation.

> Christine: I don't like him, I'm glad he's dead.

Declares her feeling.

> Therapist: It's important that you can be open with me about your thoughts and feelings concerning Tom. You can finally say you're glad he's dead. It's necessary for us to go into more details about your feelings toward Tom, especially the negative ones.

Supports patient's ability to be honest and asks for more details about her negative thoughts toward Tom.

Christine: How could he have shot me? I was so good to him and his family. He was never good to me.

Therapist: So he shoots you, you're on the ground.... As you picture this in your mind...how do you feel toward Tom?

Asks patient to relive the shooting experience and connect this with her feelings toward Tom.

Christine: I can't stand him. He's a miserable human being and crazy too...a crazy bastard.

Indicates many negative thoughts.

Therapist: And you feel...what toward him?

Pursues patient's feelings.

Christine: I'm...I guess I'm so mad at him now for what he did to me.

Declares her anger.

Therapist: Most people would feel that way. You're angry because of what he did to you. But I think there's something else going on inside you. A few moments ago you asked the question is he really dead and that you're still afraid of him.

Therapist may have moved away from the patient's angry feelings too soon. Instead, the link between Christine's fear of Tom and questions about whether he is really dead are pursued.

Christine: I am.... I wonder if he's really in the grave. I never saw him buried.

Denies Tom's death.

Therapist: So part of you thinks he's still alive and can still hurt you...as in the dream.

Clarification.

Christine: It's like I can't get away from him. Maybe if I saw him dead....

Suggests a solution.

> Therapist: Have you given any thought to going to Tom's grave?
> Sometimes it helps people to recognize that someone has
> died if they see where the person is buried.

Offers a concrete plan in the form of homework.

> Christine: The cemetery isn't far away. I could probably get my
> mother to go with me.

The therapist encourages the patient to visit the cemetery so that Tom's
death can become a reality. When she can fully accept that Tom is dead, the
mourning process can begin.

Session 8

> Christine: You're going to be happy when I tell you what I did. I
> went to the cemetery and saw Tom's grave. It's really there.
> I felt terrible.... I started to cry.

Christine begins the session by informing the therapist that she visited
Tom's grave. This indicates that she is highly motivated to work out her
complex feelings and conflicts in an active and adaptive manner. It also
demonstrates that the therapeutic alliance is positive, since she carried out
the therapist's suggestion. Nevertheless, Christine's compliance may be related to her need to be pleasing, which should be explored.

> Therapist: It's good that you went. Now you know Tom is really
> dead. You have a lot of feelings about his death.

The therapist is supportive of the patient's adaptive activity, but does
not comment about her attempt to please the therapist. At this point in
treatment, the therapist views Christine's compliance as an indicator of a
positive therapeutic relationship but recognizes that her compliance will
have to be addressed later in therapy. If this is not done, the patient's habitual character style of subservience to others will remain, and she runs the
risk of becoming a victim again.

> Christine: I don't know what I feel.... I was crying, but then
> I think about the way he treated me, and I get mad. I also
> know he did love me. Maybe that's why he shot himself.

Indicates mixed feelings toward Tom.

> Therapist: These are complex thoughts and feelings going
> through your mind. You feel sad about his death and think
> he loved you, but you also feel afraid and angry about his
> brutal way of treating you and his attempt to kill you.

Clarifies Christine's mixed feelings toward Tom.

For the remainder of this session and the next several sessions, the therapist continued to explore Tom's attempted murder of her, Christine's fear of Tom, the reality of his death, and her thought that he killed himself for her. The therapist encouraged her to mourn his death by discussing his suicide and recounting aspects of their time together. This helped her express negative feelings of anger toward Tom without thinking she was a murderer, but rather that he almost murdered her. Gradually, Christine's feelings of guilt and responsibility for Tom's suicide eased as she came to understand that his treatment of her was not really love. A well-related and empathic therapist fosters a positive therapeutic relationship, providing a basis for change.

Throughout therapy there is an ongoing educational process, which is particularly important in supportive psychotherapy. During the course of treatment, the patient identifies with the therapist and begins to incorporate aspects of the therapist's attitudes and values. Christine understood that she was not a murderer, and as a result, her feelings of guilt diminished. Her self-esteem is further enhanced by the therapist's positive regard for her. This circular process enables the patient to integrate the emotional and cognitive spheres of her life.

In Session 11, exploration of Christine's need to please became a major focus of treatment. Examination of her need to please Tom, her parents, her boss, and the therapist was undertaken in some detail. The patient was given homework assignments to keep a journal of her attempts to satisfy others while ignoring her own needs and wishes. She was helped to identify her automatic thoughts of "I must please others, or they will not like me" or "If I speak my mind, others will retaliate," then to test the logic of these assumptions and to develop better coping strategies. One of the approaches used is assertiveness training. As discussed in Chapter 5, an important issue is helping patients differentiate between assertion, passivity, and aggression. Christine's automatic thoughts were examined, and she was encouraged to change passive maladaptive behavior to assertive behavior. The next step was examination of what Christine believed to be the positive and negative consequences of being more assertive. Finally, role playing was used, and the patient was asked to assert herself with her boss and then with her father.

Case 3: Expressive–Supportive Psychotherapy— Sarah's Choice

In the initial phase of therapy, Sarah's habitual characterological pattern emerged. She believed that others, including her mother, boss, husband, and the therapist, either ignored, disappointed, or abandoned her or treated others better. For Sarah, strains in the therapeutic alliance are and will likely continue to be a common occurrence. Therefore, the therapist must continually monitor the therapeutic relationship so that ruptures in the alliance are explored and repaired. Because Sarah's treatment is on the expressive side of the continuum, her wish for a more "social" treatment approach was not gratified, but instead was explored. Finally, Sarah's pathological grief was explored, although details about her traumatic experiences in the concentration camp remained in the background until the midphase of treatment.

Session 10

In this session, the patient reacted to an unforeseen event in the therapist's office with frustration and anger. Sarah was upset because the water was turned off in the office. As a result, an exploration of the patient's thoughts and feelings toward the therapist was undertaken, which led to memories of past humiliation and deprivation.

> Sarah: Your bathroom sink is broken. I can't get any water. Oh. I was so looking forward to drinking your water. In my office, it's rusty...not clean, like yours.... I always have good water here.... I'm so thirsty.

Expresses disappointment and indicates that she looks forward to the therapist's water, implying that she obtains something good from the therapist.

> Therapist: So you're not getting good things from me. What are you feeling toward me?

Clarifies and explores Sarah's feeling.

> Sarah: There's no continuity in my life. No neighborliness.... A package was delivered yesterday and no one was home, my neighbor wouldn't accept it. I had to go to the post office.

Adaptive context is that Sarah thinks she cannot rely on anyone.

> Therapist: You're upset, I can see that, but you're not telling me what you feel about not getting water here today.

Confronts avoidance of feeling in empathic manner.

> Sarah: I'm thirsty and I'm angry with you. It's a physical need and you didn't give it to me (*yells at therapist*). You just don't have a personal interest in me!

Expresses anger in a direct manner.

> Therapist: You're angry with me because you think I'm not interested in you.

Clarifies.

> Sarah: If you really cared about me, you would have put water there...maybe in a pitcher. I feel so angry at you.... Who am I? You don't regard me as a person.

Catastrophizes situation and reacts with anger.

> Therapist: You're very angry at me; how do you experience your anger?

Explores Sarah's experience of anger.

> Sarah: I'm furious with you *(face reddened)*. You could have gotten water.

> Therapist: I see your point, but why would you think that not having water means I don't regard you as a person?

Acknowledges Sarah's need but confronts her overreaction to the situation, which reflects Sarah's inability to integrate cognitive and emotional responses.

> Sarah: I thought you didn't want to give me water.

Cognitive distortion. Attributes willful withholding by therapist.

> Therapist: Why would I withhold water? In fact, the water was just turned off for repairs in the building, but you have a point. It would've been better if I had been able to get some bottled water.

Provides explanation to correct Sarah's cognitive distortion, but acknowledges the reality of the situation.

> Sarah: I should be able to control physical functions. I'm ashamed...I reacted so much.

Connects thirst to bodily functions with shame.

> Therapist: What are you ashamed about?

Sarah: I'm embarrassed with every bodily function...defecating, urinating, being thirsty or hungry. It's humiliating. When I was in the camp, I lost control. I had to go to the bathroom, I was sick. The *Kapo* [an inmate in charge of a work team] wouldn't let me go. I had diarrhea. This was the hardest to bear, not thirst.

Deprivation of water leads to Sarah's concentration camp experiences.

Therapist: What can I say, that must have been horrible.... Tell me what's going on in your mind now.

Empathizes and explores.

Sarah: I don't know if you are aware of how it was. We were in bunks, one over the other. When I couldn't control my diarrhea, it dripped on her, whoever was on the bottom. It was a tragedy to the girl under me.

Describes loss of control of bodily function and its effect on others.

Therapist: And for you, too.

Empathically focuses on Sarah.

Sarah: I should be able to do the impossible.

Unrealistic expectation for total control.

Therapist: No, I don't think so. How could you have control over your bodily functions when you were so ill at times and at the mercy of the guards?

Reality-tests with support.

Sarah: I...for a bite of bread, I was dependent. I always tried to anticipate what people wanted. I was with a group, we were seven people. I trusted them that they wouldn't do anything to hurt me, but when there was a vacancy...in a better place...I didn't think twice about leaving them, I had no loyalty. I wasn't *disloyal*, but I left them.

Describes ability to behave in accordance with reality and raises questions concerning her commitment to others. Linkage to mother, Doreen, Ernest, and the therapist? What was adaptive in the concentration camp may no longer be adaptive.

Therapist: So when the opportunity arose, you made choices that enabled you to survive. You had the strength to make some hard choices and did the best you could, would you agree?

Reassures, affirms, and admires.

Sarah: Yes, I tried to stay alive for my father. If he found out about my mother and the family, he wouldn't want to live. I had to stay alive for him. The *Kapo* chose me to be with a group where there were special home-type things to do, like sewing and cleaning. The *Kapo*'s sister was a cook, and she had a son my age...she did things for me. The top of the soup was water, the bottom had potatoes; she gave me from the bottom.

Describes how others helped her.

Therapist: So when I didn't have water today, you believed I intentionally turned it off. Being deprived when you were in the concentration camp was calculated, and inhumane, but today it just happened by chance. Your thinking was correct and adaptive back then, but now you're thinking in the same way, having the same kind of thought with me.

Describes Sarah's dysfunctional thinking.

Sarah: *(Laughs)* It's ridiculous...idiotic...but I think yes.... It is like I'm thinking in the past, not now.

Agrees.

Therapist: So, what was once true is no longer true, even though you are sometimes convinced it is, like today, when you feel deprived of water.

Emphasizes difference between past and present.

Sarah: When I feel deprived, I think I'm being written off as a person.

Deprivation leads to loss of self-esteem (in the past for Sarah, loss of life).

Therapist: What about here with me? How does it apply?

Focuses on therapeutic relationship.

Sarah: I didn't know what to make of it. I feel a regard for me as a person by you...not passing a verdict over me. There was no one to complain to until now. I had to put it all on ice (*laughs*).

Senses therapist's regard and expresses positive view of therapist.

Therapist: On that note, since we're having a thaw, let's see how this kind of experience with me occurs with other people in your life. We know you've had similar experiences with Ernest and Doreen, where you felt written off as a person.

Links rupture in the therapeutic alliance with husband and supervisor.

Sarah: With Ernest it happens all the time. I told you what happened with the insurance agent. Ernest dismissed me. He said he had business things to talk to him about and that I should leave them alone.

Easily gives an example, indicating the alliance rupture has been repaired.

Therapist: How did you feel about being excluded?

Pursues affect.

Sarah: I was furious at Ernest.

Expresses feeling easily and directly.

Therapist: What did you do about it?

Asks for behavioral response.

Sarah: Nothing. I left the room. Later, I told him I didn't like it. He thought I was ridiculous. He said, "Why would you be interested, it was just business." I was so angry I walked out of the room and wouldn't talk to him.

Angrily withdraws from conflict.

Therapist: So you were furious with him, but instead of standing up for yourself and letting Ernest know what you thought, you became passive and left the room.

Confronts Sarah's passivity.

Sarah: It wouldn't do any good to say anything, so I just gave up.

Maintains passive stance.

> Therapist: Giving up is one choice; there are others, like standing up for yourself. If Ernest was standing here now, what would you want to say to him?

Asks patient to practice being more active and assertive.

> Sarah: Uh...Oh, this is ridiculous...I guess I'd say, "From now on, I want to stay when business is going on that involves me. I'm not a child" *(cries).*

Halfheartedly stands up for herself.

> Therapist: Okay, but remember you tend to walk away and leave when you think it's your only choice—the way you also did with Doreen when she neglected to recommend you for a promotion.

Restates Sarah's maladaptive behavior.

> Sarah: I don't like hearing this...I'd rather walk away—who needs to struggle? I don't need it.

Continues her passive position.

> Therapist: It's hard to make changes, but you have a choice. You can leave things as they are and walk away from conflict, or you can begin to stand up for yourself in a way that makes sense, so that your relationships can change.

Continues to confront Sarah's defensive withdrawal while presenting a more adaptive solution.

> Sarah: I guess you're right, but it's not easy to change the way I am. I get so angry.

In this session, a rupture in the therapeutic alliance occurred when the patient accused the therapist of intentionally withholding water based on her belief that people sought to deprive and exclude her. Although there was some justification for her complaint, Sarah's tendency to catastrophize overrode the reality of the situation, which stemmed from her early life and concentration camp experiences. When her anger at the therapist did not meet with retaliation, the misalliance was repaired. The therapist went on to link this experience in the therapeutic relationship to similar conflicts with Sarah's husband and former boss. In the next few sessions, the therapist continued to explore these relationships and connected these experiences with earlier relationships with her mother and father.

Session 12

> Sarah: I'm furious at Ernest.
>
> Therapist: What about?
>
> Sarah: After dinner he said, "Do you want to do the dishes, or should I?" What kind of thing is that to say? What does that mean? I was furious.

Appears to be a misappraisal of Ernest's question.

> Therapist: You were furious with Ernest; what was it like?

Explores affect first, another option might have been to address Sarah's dysfunctional thinking.

> Sarah: I was burning up. I felt like walking out, but this time I didn't. I just held it in and didn't talk to him for a few hours.

Openly expresses anger, but indicates that she remained in a silent fury with Ernest.

> Therapist: What were you thinking?

Addresses thinking.

> Sarah: I'm always looking for hidden meaning. He didn't want to do the dishes. I'm always left to do the work—cooking, cleaning, and everything.

Reveals automatic thought of "Even though he asked the question, he didn't want to do the dishes."

> Therapist: So, you wanted Ernest to tell you he would do the dishes, yet you told me you said nothing for several hours. How could he know what you wanted if you didn't tell him?

Addresses automatic thinking.

Sarah: He should know what to do, I am not required to tell him. I always feel obligated to do what the other person wants. I try to anticipate and please others; can't he anticipate what I want?

Wants husband to automatically understand and meet her needs.

Therapist: So you have mixed feelings. You want to please Ernest on the one hand, and on the other you want him to please you and to anticipate what you need or want.

Clarifies Sarah's needs.

Sarah: Wants are not allowed.... Even when I was a little girl, I wasn't supposed to ask for what I wanted.

Moves to past and indicates that this represents a long-term conflict.

Therapist: That's important, we'll get to it, but let's stay with your thoughts and feelings about Ernest now. You're in a tough spot with Ernest if wants aren't allowed, because you don't tell him what you want and then you get furious at him for not supplying what you need. What do you think?

Brings Sarah back to conflict with Ernest and clarifies conflict. The therapist is working within the triangles of conflict and person. In the triangle of conflict, Sarah has an unexpressed need/wish that is defended against with anger and withdrawal. In the triangle of the person, this response is directed toward a current person in her life (husband).

Sarah: Asking is hard for me.

Therapist: Yes, I know, but you're attributing hidden meaning to Ernest's question about the dishes. One possibility is that he was asking you to tell him what you wanted. If you told him you wanted him to do the dishes, what would have happened?

Addresses Sarah's dysfunctional thinking.

Sarah: Well...if you put it that way *(smiles)*, I guess he would have done the dishes.

Indicates that it may be possible to change her thinking.

There was further exploration of another incident involving Ernest and their children in which the patient had felt unimportant and rejected, leading her to become angry with and withdraw from her husband. The therapist then turned to the past.

> Therapist: A few minutes ago you mentioned that when you were a little girl, you weren't supposed to ask for anything, so you're indicating that this kind of conflict goes back to your childhood.

> Sarah: I'm trying to move ahead, but it's so hard. I'm afraid to take chances. I have lots of thoughts about not being deserving. When I was a little girl, I was told that I was only a child. It was spelled out for me that whatever it is, I don't deserve it.

Indicates that her needs were not considered.

> Therapist: So not feeling deserving or having your needs met goes back to when you were a little girl, and now you automatically think everyone will treat you the same way.

Explains automatic thought as developing earlier and continuing in her present life.

> Sarah: My mother believed that children had no rights.

> Therapist: You wanted Ernest to care about you and do something for you; what did you want from your mother?

Explores Sarah's wish.

> Sarah: I was never considered. What I wanted was unimportant.

Defensive avoidance.

> Therapist: It must be difficult for you to answer the question of what you wanted from your mother, because you move away from it.

Confronts Sarah's avoidance in an empathic manner.

> Sarah: I wanted her to care about me (*eyes begin to fill with tears*).

Expresses wish.

> Therapist: I notice tears in your eyes. What are you experiencing?

Points out nonverbal behavior and asks Sarah to elaborate.

> Sarah: I didn't really want her to leave me in the concentration camp. If she'd cared, she would have come with me, not my sisters. I didn't have enough time with her.

Sarah may also be referring to her time with the therapist.

> Therapist: You're right. Your time with your mother was cut short.

When working with individuals with multiple traumas, it is often necessary to return to an exploration of past experiences throughout therapy. This promotes the working-through process leading to behavioral change.

This session illustrates the use of dynamic and cognitive techniques in an integrated approach. The therapist was able to explore Sarah's conflict with Ernest and to link it to a similar conflict with her mother. At the same time, the therapist highlighted Sarah's cognitive distortions so that her automatic thoughts would yield to reality.

Session 14

The patient enters the office 7 minutes late.

> Sarah: *(Silence at first)* I'm feeling good; maybe I don't need therapy anymore.

Three bits of information are offered by Sarah: she is late, she is feeling good, and she believes she may not need treatment any more.

> Therapist: Tell me about the good feeling.

Chooses to explore the good feeling to assess readiness for termination.

> Sarah: Well, remember I told you I thought my boss, Martin, was annoyed at me for going to the dentist and coming in late.

Brings up lateness. (Sarah had started a new job the week before).

> Therapist: Yes, what about it?

Explores.

> Sarah: He wasn't mad. I was wrong. He likes my work, and I enjoy working in this office; it uses my brain.

Describes positive response from boss which may lead to a change in automatic thinking.

Therapist: Sounds good, work is going well and your negative expectation about Martin's reaction to your lateness was unfounded. Speaking of lateness, what happened today?

Clarifies Sarah's thinking and confronts her lateness.

Sarah: I lost track of time and I left work late.

Therapist: I wonder how you thought I would react to your lateness?

Using a dynamic framework, the therapist is asking for Sarah's fantasy; in a cognitive approach, this would be considered a probe of Sarah's thinking.

Sarah: *(Pause)* I was thinking that you would be upset with me.

Describes automatic thought.

Therapist: By upset, you mean...?

Sarah: Annoyed...I thought you wouldn't like it.

Therapist: You thought I would be annoyed with you, and you came in wanting to stop treatment with me. Is there a connection?

Clarifies and links wish to stop treatment with lateness (interprets).

Sarah: As I told you before, I always try to anticipate others' reactions.

Confirms interpretation and connects it to past behavior.

Therapist: And how did I react?

Asks Sarah to test her dysfunctional thought.

Sarah: You don't seem angry.

Therapist: So this thought is coming from your experience with other people in your life. What do you think? With Martin you realized your expectation was faulty, and with Ernest you had a similar experience.

Connects Sarah's dysfunctional thinking with other persons in her life. From a dynamic perspective, the therapist is using the triangle of the person to link Sarah's experience in the patient-therapist relationship with other significant people in her life.

Sarah: It's the way I am. I expect a certain reaction. I used to get angry at my mother and tell her I was running away. When I said that, she sent me outside and told me to wait, and she went back into the house, packed up a bag, and told me to go into the world and run away. Then she locked the door. I was scared. How could I let her win? I was in her power. I wanted her to stop me.

Offers a memory of running away and not being stopped by mother. May be an allusion to termination.

Therapist: You wanted her to stop you. What would it mean to you if she had stopped you?

Explores underlying wish.

Sarah: I always wanted her to love me. I wanted her to care for me no matter what I did. If she had stopped me, I would have known she loved me.

Expresses wish for mother's love.

Therapist: It's clear that you wanted your mother's love and often felt that she didn't give you enough.

Clarifies Sarah's wish.

Sarah: It was confusing to me, because sometimes I got a lot of attention from her.

Therapist: When was that?

Sarah: When my father was away on business, she used to take me into her bed at night and we slept together. When he came home, she made me leave the bed.

Retells story of closeness with mother which was interrupted by father.

Therapist: How did you feel toward your mother when she took you into her bed?

The therapist chose to focus on Sarah's positive feelings for her mother. It may have been preferable to explore Sarah's negative feelings toward her father for coming between them and toward her mother for choosing her father. This was worked on during a later session.

> Sarah: I loved to be with her. I felt she really cared about me, and I felt close to her. When my father was there, I wanted to stay with both of them.

Indicates wish for both mother and father.

> Therapist: So you've always expected to be pushed out or eventually not treated well. Could this be related to your tendency to expect a negative response from people, as we saw with me, Ernest, and Martin?

Interprets rejection by parents as underlying current negative expectation. Utilizing the triangle of conflict, Sarah's wish (W) was to receive love from her parents. Her response was to become angry and withdraw (defense). In the triangle of the person, this conflict with her parents was linked to current figures in her life and to the therapist.

> Sarah: I expect criticism and rejection. I guess I don't really think about it.

Confirms interpretation.

> Therapist: When you were a child with your parents you were relatively powerless, but now as an adult it's different. You didn't have a lot of choices back then. Now you're in a position to make choices, make your wishes known, and stand up for yourself in a good way.

The midphase of therapy for Sarah consisted of working through her conflicts and dysfunctional thinking. The therapist connected the conflicts with current figures and in the here and now of the therapeutic relationship to similar conflicts with her parents. In turn, the conflicts with Sarah's parents were linked to current figures and to the therapist. These connections are part of the circular process of working through conflicts to achieve insight and behavioral change. New insights and behavioral change can lead to further resolution of conflicts.

Case 4: Expressive Psychotherapy— The Man Who Never Said Goodbye

The work of uncovering during the initial phase of treatment proceeded in a fairly smooth manner. For Mark, a relatively high-functioning individual, the midphase of psychotherapy will involve working through. The multiple losses he sustained in the past must be connected to his current behavior and to aspects of the therapeutic relationship. In addition, continued cognitive restructuring needs to be done to promote mastery of Mark's impulsive behavior.

Session 14

> Mark: I'm having trouble at work. It's hard for me to do what they expect from me. We are losing a lot of money...they want me to make changes.... I've been developing a number of new methodologies, but the way Elliot *(supervisor)* wants to do it is not working. It's hard for me to deal with him...I have to get a different job. My father-in-law has a possible job for me with a company he does business with. I don't like the kind of work they do, but I can't talk to my father-in-law about it.

The adaptive context of this session is Mark's passivity toward his supervisor and father-in-law.

> Therapist: So there's something about this company you don't like, but you aren't able to talk to your father-in-law about it...what is his name?

Clarifies and asks for first name.

> Mark: Charles. I get along with him. But, when he's in a bad mood, he can be nasty...not to me, though.

> Therapist: What kind of man is Charles?

Asks for description of Charles in order to make him come alive in the therapy.

> Mark: He's strong and robust. He's a dominating man...big.

> Therapist: And when you're with him, how do you feel?

> Mark: Not dominated...I feel gratitude and kindly and loving toward him. He can be nasty to Sue or the opposite. I see these things as something that always will pass. He is generous, thinking, and caring.

Expresses mixed feelings for Charles.

> Therapist: So you have a lot of positive feelings for Charles while recognizing his foibles.

Clarification.

> Mark: Yes, but it's hard for me to talk with him. I didn't get back to him after he told me about the job. I guess he's waiting.

Describes his passivity.

> Therapist: So you're holding back, not bringing up your concerns about the job with Charles. In the face of these concerns, you become passive with him and don't act in a positive way to get yourself a new job.

Confronts Mark's passivity.

> Mark: Yes, I could be pushing for myself and getting a better job, but the job is with a company that manufactures parts for rockets. I'm afraid of it.

> Therapist: Afraid?

> Mark: I'm afraid I'll owe this to Charles…to do well since he's helping me to get the job. I feel a pull to please him…. It's a strong motivation. When I did well in business school, he would praise me…be proud of me…support me.

Fear of neediness.

> Therapist: So he is sort of like a parent, a father to you.

Clarification.

> Mark: Exactly.

> Therapist: And your feelings about this, about Charles?

> Mark: *(Laughs)* I shouldn't need to feel like I need a father, but I do.

Defensive laughter.

> Therapist: You're laughing…. What are you experiencing?

Confronts defense.

> Mark: Here I am getting older…I want to be on my own and strong, and I'm so focused on having a father.

Highlights conflictual wishes; the need for a parental figure versus the wish to feel self-sufficient and strong.

> Therapist: You have a wish to have a helpful, powerful father and you also want to be on your own, making your own decisions. So you avoid Charles.

Interprets conflict.

> Mark: Sue's father is the kind of person with whom I've had this need. Now if I open this up with him, I'll be pursuing him.

> Therapist: What's the problem with pursuing him?

Explores.

> Mark: Well, I don't know... everyone looks for their pound of flesh.

Fears Charles will take something from him.

> Therapist: We know people have disappointed you, especially men...your father, brother, previous therapist...and with me, earlier in treatment...so you don't fully trust Charles.

Interprets Mark's disappointment with a number of men.

> Mark: Yes, but I know Charles is not like that...but I can't let him help me.

Persists in avoidance.

> Therapist: In the face of this conflict, you become passive. We know you fall back on two sorts of extreme ways of behaving...either you become passive or you have a temper tantrum. With Charles you become passive, you put him off, but you end up defeating yourself.

Repeats interpretation of Mark's habitual behavior, in which he alternates between passivity and temper tantrums and ends in self-sabotage.

> Mark: I see that. I try to defeat myself a lot.

> Therapist: We have also seen this with me (previous session) and with other men in your life—your father, your brother—and with Charles.

Links patient-therapist relationship with father, brother, and Charles.

In this session, the therapist was able to interpret Mark's maladaptive ways of behaving with either passivity or temper tantrums. The underlying wish to have a loving, caring parent clearly emerged, which may be an allusion to the therapist. At the same time, Mark is fearful of losing his autonomy and perhaps bodily integrity (in a classical psychoanalytic framework, this would be understood as castration anxiety).

Session 15

> Mark: Last night my daughter Liz woke up. She was crying and frightened, so I sat with her awhile. When I walked out, she started screaming. She woke me from a dream. Something happened at work that upset me. A young woman was let go who was about to be married. The day before, my boss gave a toast to her at an office party... it was a toast to her for success in her marriage. The dream was meaningful.... In the dream, I'm with my boss and my daughter Liz is on my lap. I'm embarrassed in front of my boss. I guess I wanted Elliot to hold me and be a father like I am a father to Liz.

Continues to express a wish for a caring father.

> Therapist: So the dream indicated that you're wanting a father, someone to care about you, and also someone to love.

Clarifies.

> Mark: Yes... after the dream... the next day, Elliot asked all of us in our group what we thought about a presentation he gave. I said, "It addressed the issues," but I don't really know if he did it successfully. Everything he showed indicated that we're the best! After I said I thought he addressed the issues, he put his hand on my shoulder in a friendly way. Later I met Fran (colleague) in the hall. She moved past me quickly, maybe she knows I'm fired. Elliot, who gave the toast... fired the woman he toasted the next day. And I see him as a father.

Elaborates conflict of wanting a caring father, while fearing rejection.

> Therapist: So you want Elliot to be a father to you, but you're afraid he'll let you go.

Interprets conflict.

Mark: I see that, I can't trust anyone.

Therapist: How does that apply to me?

Looks for a similar conflict in patient-therapist relationship.

Mark: I see you as a kind of parent...father.

Therapist: You see Elliot as a kind of father and are afraid he'll let you go.... Do you have a similar concern about me?

Continues to focus on conflict in therapeutic relationship.

Mark: *(Laughs)* Well, this therapy has to end, so you will let me go.

Confirms transference interpretation.

Therapist: What's that like for you?

Explores.

Mark: I know we talked about this before and I don't like it...I wish it could be different, but I do feel you're kind. You're helpful to me without using jargon. You help me focus on real issues...I've never looked at my anger like I do here. One thing a boy looks to his father for is to help him with his problems, but I don't really know you.

States negative feelings about time-limited therapy and positive regard for therapist, but suggests he would like to know therapist better.

Therapist: You would like to know me better?

Clarifies.

Mark: Yes. I'd like to be a fly on the wall, observe you, really know you.

Therapist: So you have a yearning to be close with me...a closeness that you don't remember with your father. How would you have liked it to have been with your father?

Interprets wish for closeness with therapist and links this to father. It might have been preferable to remain within the here and now of the therapeutic relationship and to make the link to the father later. The shift to Mark's father may have been based on the therapist's discomfort with the yearning expressed by Mark.

> Mark: I have too many angry feelings toward my father. I never talked about this. Everyone always thought he was an insignificant person in my life, because I was so young when he died.

Moves to anger toward father rather than closeness.

> Therapist: Do you remember some experiences with him?

Asks for concrete examples of relationship with father.

> Mark: Since I've been seeing you, my memory for things is much better. I remember things.... He brought home his secretary... She looked good...made a fuss about me.... I enjoyed that.

Reflects a therapeutic alliance.

> Therapist: So this is a pleasant memory not associated with anger.

Clarifies.

> Mark: But why did it take this stranger to get my father to notice me? It annoys me. My father was playing a role...and was really not giving anything to me.

Expresses anger toward father.

> Therapist: So you felt he was withholding.

> Mark: Not only with me, he didn't give to my brother or mother. I wanted recognition.... Growing up, I wanted him to value me so I could value myself.

Indicates self-esteem suffered from father's withholding.

> Therapist: You wanted your father to value you?

> Mark: I wanted recognition, I wanted to know that he loved me. You asked me what I think of you. You're interested in me... you care...it's something I didn't get from my father.

Links father and therapist in contrasting ways.

Therapist: You wanted love, kindness and support from your father. He died and this cut you off from him.

Raises death of father.

Mark: I can remember feeling jealous when my brother came home from college. He showed his college ring, and my father was interested. I wanted my father to be interested in me.

Therapist: We're talking about your feeling that you didn't get your father's interest, and last week we didn't meet. It occurs to me that maybe you have some feelings about that.

Recognizes something is not being addressed in the patient-therapist relationship.

Mark: Yes. I missed you. It's hard for me to deal with this.

Therapist: In what way?

Mark: I can't tell you what a special time this is for me...not feeling any guilt.... I can rely on you. You make my world better...you're unique in my life.

Expresses strong positive feelings for therapist.

Therapist: You're having strong feelings about me. I see you're getting tears in your eyes.

Clarifies and highlights Mark's nonverbal behavior (tears).

Mark: I feel very strongly...a lot like I want to hug you.

Mark continued the theme from the previous session, relating his wish to be cared for and loved. His fear of rejection was explored, which led to his expression of positive feelings for the therapist. The therapist linked this to his father, and the patient brought up his wish to have had a loving relationship with his father. However, he believed that his father had been withholding, which led Mark to express anger toward him. The session closed with the patient expressing warm and tender feelings about the therapist. This constitutes a corrective emotional experience for Mark that can serve as a bridge in his relationships, both past and present. At the same time, the therapist had some countertransferential difficulties with being the focus of Mark's loving feelings.

Conclusions

The midphase of treatment is characterized by a structure-building, problem-solving, and/or working-through process. In this chapter we presented the continued treatment of Lucy, Christine, Sarah, and Mark. For each patient, the therapeutic work was individually tailored on the basis of their placement on the psychotherapy continuum. For Lucy, who is on the supportive side of the continuum, the emphasis was on cognitive restructuring, problem solving, and education about her illness and her need for medication. With Christine, the techniques used were also supportive and contained some expressive elements. Cognitive-behavioral techniques such as exposure therapy, identifying and exploring automatic thoughts, and homework were essential in the midphase of Christine's treatment. Sarah, on the expressive side of the continuum, was treated with exploratory psychotherapy as well as cognitive-behavioral and supportive techniques, which helped her work through conflicts and traumas. Mark's treatment was predominately expressive. The working-through process for Mark consisted of connecting important people in his life, both past and present, with the therapist. Transference interpretations served to produce insight and to set the stage for later behavioral change.

CHAPTER

9

Termination
Phase of Treatment

When patient and therapist are ending their journey together and the end is in sight, they will need to say goodbye to one another. The personal meaning each brings to the relationship will determine how the process of termination unfolds. Ending treatment may be fraught with a range of problems, conflicts, thoughts, feelings, and behaviors which will need to be considered.

For most people, saying goodbye is not easy. An individual's experience with attachment, separation, and loss will play a major role in the termination process. Patients who have experienced significant losses may have a hard time ending treatment. For them, ending with the therapist will evoke memories and the associated thoughts and feelings about earlier losses. In this sense, termination is analogous to a mourning process.

At the same time, the patient's position on the psychological structure/psychotherapy continuum will determine the relative amounts of exploration and support the therapist will use. In more expressive therapy, the loss of the therapist must be worked through and connected to previous losses. The loss of the therapist presents an opportunity to explore and work out losses of significant people in the patient's life by using the here and now of the therapeutic relationship as a vehicle to make the process come alive with affect. In supportive psychotherapy, less emphasis is placed on the past, and losses are worked through in a cognitive manner; affective experiencing is not stressed. Adaptation, psychological functioning, and self-esteem are monitored, supported, and strengthened, as always, throughout the termination phase.

Patients who have not sustained significant losses or who have effectively worked them through will experience the termination process without a great deal of conflict or difficulty. For them, the number of sessions needed for termination will be relatively few. Indeed, some patients rightly view ending treatment as an accomplishment and recognize that they have improved significantly and have achieved their goals.

It should be recognized that for some severely impaired patients, termination should not be considered.

> A 38-year-old man with a diagnosis of chronic schizophrenia and a history of six hospitalizations was treated with supportive psychotherapy and medication. He improved enough so that his major symptoms diminished and he was able to return to work. However, he still required a great deal of support in activities of daily living and medication maintenance. His therapy sessions were gradually reduced to once a month.

It would not be advisable to stop treatment with this patient, even if he continued to improve. Treatment frequency could be further reduced to every 3 or 4 months or less. Many patients with this degree of pathology should be considered lifetime patients.

Patients with personality disorder generally will terminate in a way that is consistent with their character patterns. Individuals with major dependency needs will often require a longer period of termination, and the process will be more complicated. With these patients, the therapist must begin to work on separation and termination early on. Transference will often be intense, and the therapist may experience countertransference reactions based on the patient's neediness (see Chapter 4). On the other hand, patients who use a great deal of denial or avoidance may terminate quickly and deny difficulty separating from the therapist.

A number of questions naturally arise concerning termination. How is the decision made about when to terminate treatment, and who decides? Is termination final, or can the patient freely contact the therapist at a later time? If the treating clinician is a psychiatrist and medication is part of the treatment, how is the transition to a medication maintenance phase accomplished?

The idea to end treatment may originate with either member of the dyad. When there is mutual agreement, the termination process is set in motion. At this point, the therapist can suggest that they undertake a review of the progress made in treatment. A useful approach is to reassess each of the patient's areas of disturbance or target complaints (Battle et al. 1966) to determine how much progress has been made and what, if anything, remains to be accomplished. Numerical ratings of each target complaint can be compared with the initial scoring during the evaluation process or descriptive accounts can be obtained from patients.

The length of time needed for termination will vary, depending on many of the issues discussed above. Some patients will terminate quickly and easily in just a few sessions, while others with significant loss issues or dependency needs may require more time. Termination need not be thought of as fixed and final. We believe in an open-door policy in which patients are free to call or come back if or when the need arises.

Case 1: Supportive Psychotherapy— The Woman Who Lived on the Edge

By the fifteenth session, Lucy indicated that she was feeling much better. Her adaptation and psychological (ego) functioning had improved. She was able to care for herself and her children, and she had stopped pursuing her abusive boyfriend. Her relationship with the therapist remained positive throughout the therapy.

Session 15

> Therapist: How is it going?
>
> Lucy: Last week I went back to work. People were glad to see me. Joanne, she works with me, brought coffee and doughnuts, you know...like a welcome-back breakfast.... I guess everyone chipped in...never expected it.

Indicates that she has gone back to work and received a positive reception from co-workers.

> Therapist: So everyone was glad to see you, and they held a welcome-back party for you.

Restatement.

Lucy: I know…some people called while I was out, they wanted to know how I was and when I was coming back… *(shrugs shoulders)*.

Therapist: You didn't expect your co-workers to be so welcoming, and to miss you. What's it like for you to know that Joanne and the others were interested in you while you were on maternity leave and now are celebrating your return to work?

Supports self-esteem.

Lucy: Good, it really felt good.

Therapist: So you felt surprised and pleased by the special breakfast.

Lucy: I didn't know they were going to do that…. They really prepared. And someone made a sign. It said "Welcome back, Lucy."

Therapist: So, thinking about all of this and your view of yourself, don't you think that others, your co-workers, value you and are pleased to be with you?

Continues to support self-esteem.

Lucy: Yes, I got embarrassed by all the attention, but it made me feel good…. At home I thought about it. They gave me a gift for Crystal, a little bench with her name on it.

Therapist: It's really wonderful that the good feeling stayed with you. What about the rest of your life?

The therapist continues to assess how Lucy is doing. If the patient is no longer depressed or anxious and is functioning well, session frequency can be reduced and the patient can enter a maintenance phase of treatment, either with a psychiatrist or with a primary care physician. Because Lucy has a history of severe recurrent depressions and panic as well as interpersonal problems, her current therapist, a psychiatrist, will continue to monitor her medication.

Lucy: For the past few weeks I've been managing pretty okay.

Acknowledges improvement.

Therapist: Let's look at that. Tell me about Crystal and Brenda.

Moves from general to specific.

> Lucy: The baby is sleeping through the night now most of the time, so taking care of her is okay. She's even starting to hold the bottle, the small water bottle. I'm glad I had her...and the baby-sitter is a nice woman...and good with the baby and Brenda, too.

> Therapist: And Brenda, how is she doing?

> Lucy: Well, she doesn't talk too much, but she's doing her homework better, and when I came home yesterday, I saw the baby-sitter helping her with math.... I was glad I didn't have to do it.

> Therapist: I can understand that. You made a good choice when you hired Mrs. Hodge *(the baby-sitter)*.

Uses praise appropriately.

> Lucy: She goes to my church. She's a grandmother and she likes to keep busy.

> Therapist: So it's a mutually satisfying partnership.

> Lucy: Yeah, and I don't have to worry when I'm at work. Carl *(patient's husband)* still comes home at crazy hours, so he can't help too much.

Raises a continuing problem.

> Therapist: So you can work with a clear mind, but how are you handling Carl's erratic hours?

Explores Lucy's coping ability.

> Lucy: I feel sorry for him. He works hard and he pays for almost everything. He would do anything for Brenda, and I think Crystal too.

Recognizes positives about Carl in relation to the children.

> Therapist: What about your relationship with Carl? We've talked about it. Are things progressing since he came here with you?

Refocuses Lucy on Carl.

Lucy: We are talking more. It's still hard for me to say what I want, and I still don't like how much he works.

Therapist: What would you say if it was easier for you to be freer with Carl?

Asks Lucy to practice saying what she wants from Carl.

Lucy: I want more affection, but it's more like a brother and sister thing with us.

Declares her need.

Therapist: Why not tell Carl you want more affection?

Encourages Lucy to be more direct.

Lucy: Maybe I'll try, but I can deal with it. He said he'll take me out on a horse-and-buggy ride in Central Park with Brenda. I need to have fun. All he thinks about is work; then he's tired. But he's a good man. I know it, and I'm doing all right now.

Therapist: So we've looked at different parts of your life, and you're doing all right now. What about your depression?

Completes survey.

Lucy: Well, I'm pretty good. No more depression...no crying... I'm sleeping well.... I'm better.

Therapist: And the panic symptoms; your heart pounding, short-ness of breath, dizziness, thinking you're going to die?

Lucy: All gone.... Sometimes I worry about it coming back, but no, it's gone. I can manage now.

Therapist: And the medication, are you doing okay with it?

Lucy: Yes, I'm taking it...two pills every morning. You know, I think I don't need to come anymore. I'm busy with lots of things now.

Able to be direct with therapist.

Therapist: So things are pretty good and I think you're right, but it doesn't make sense for you to stop coming altogether,

because we need to continue to monitor the medication to
try to make sure you don't get sick again. We can meet less often... what do you think?

Reiterates importance of medication maintenance.

Lucy: I was thinking that I don't need to come anymore....
I didn't think about the medication.

The session began with Lucy responding to the therapist's question about
how things were going with a positive response about work. Her ability to
successfully return to work was a sign that she had improved significantly.
The therapist recognized that the treatment was entering the maintenance
phase and undertook a review of the patient's major areas of disturbance.
The ease with which the patient was able to communicate with the therapist
was a marker of her improvement. She was able to handle the tasks of everyday life and to successfully care for her baby and older daughter. She had
reached an accommodation with her husband and was able to speak somewhat more directly to him and to accept the fact that his job required him to
go out of town occasionally. She described her relationship with him as more
like a brother and sister than a husband and wife. Although not ideal, the
patient felt the relationship was satisfactory. She was able to find a reliable
baby-sitter, which enabled her to return to work. In addition, she reestab-
lished ties to her church, which enlarged her social support network. This
strong support system, consisting of family, women in her church, employer,
and family doctor, is invaluable for a successful transition to medication
maintenance.

Another issue in shifting the focus of treatment is the therapist's countertransference feelings. Transitioning to medication maintenance changes
the nature of the therapeutic relationship. The therapist is less involved in
an in-depth manner and may have feelings of loss.

Session 16

Lucy began the session by describing the previous 3 weeks. She had no
symptoms or problems with the medication and continued to work, take
care of her children, and maintain a relatively satisfactory relationship with
her husband. When this review was completed, the therapist asked how
Lucy felt about coming less frequently.

Lucy: It's okay. I like talking to you, and you've helped me a lot,
but it's different now, I'm really back to myself.

Therapist: So, you feel good about yourself and our work together. Since we will be meeting less frequently, you should
feel free to call me if anything comes up, or if you have any
problems with the medication.

Supports self-esteem and indicates availability if a new problem arises.

As the transition is made to a maintenance phase of therapy, it may be
destructive to confront Lucy's defenses and thus potentially undermine
them. In addition, because this was a supportive psychotherapy, the patient's adaptive defenses should be supported and interventions raising
anxiety avoided.

Therapist: I appreciate your telling me that I was helpful. We
have a partnership, and you worked hard at getting yourself
better.

Emphasizes collaborative nature of the relationship.

Lucy: I know that. I wouldn't feel so different now if I didn't come
here.

Therapist: I enjoyed working with you for these past 4 months,
and I'll continue to see you for your medication; you should
feel free to call me if you need to talk.

At the end of the session, the therapist highlighted the patient's ongoing
need for medication and noted that they would continue to meet to monitor
the medication. The therapist indicated his availability to the patient if any
problems came up in the future. In supportive psychotherapy, it is particularly important to leave the door open so patients know they can see the
therapist if necessary. Leaving the door open maintains the therapeutic relationship and retains the therapist as an object in the patient's life.

Case 2: Supportive-Expressive Psychotherapy—
The Woman Who Thought She Was a Murderer

During the midphase of treatment, Christine was able to reexperience the
traumatic event that almost resulted in her death, to mourn the loss of Tom,
and to realize she was not responsible for his suicide. The view of herself as
a murderer gradually shifted as the therapist helped to correct cognitive distortions. Early in the mourning process, she was able to acknowledge and
express her angry feelings toward Tom. Time was spent working on Chris-

tine's thoughts and feelings about her mother and father, who did not acknowledge Tom's brutal treatment of their daughter. Christine's father was abusive to her and her siblings when they were children, so that Tom's behavior was in part a repetition of her childhood experiences with her father. For the last few sessions, the therapist has taken a more exploratory position. Christine has improved and no longer requires as much supportive work. This transition represents a shift to a midpoint on the psychopathology–psychological structure continuum.

Session 13

> Christine: My parents had a fight. I can't stand it when they start yelling. Why does my mother put up with it? She should leave him, but she never will. You'll never guess what happened after the fight.

The adaptive context in this session appears to be related to her parents and issues of separation.

> Therapist: You're probably right.

> Christine: They went to Atlantic City! One minute my mother is screaming and yelling, and the next, she's going with him to gamble.

Indicates mother accepts father's abusiveness.

> Therapist: What do you think about that?

Therapist begins to explore.

> Christine: It's crazy...my mother takes it. He never bothered with us.... He doesn't care.

Recognizes mother's passive acceptance of father's behavior and indicates that it applies to entire family.

> Therapist: So he didn't care about the whole family, but let's see how it is between you and your father.

Focuses on Christine and father and not on entire family which would be too general.

> Christine: It's pretty awful. My father is always mad, and he doesn't think of anyone but himself. Everything annoys him. Once

we were at a wedding and Tom was mad at me. My father was standing there, and he saw Tom pull me out of the place we were in…my father just stood there. I said, "Dad"; my father just looked mad and walked away. When Tom got me outside, he slapped me, he said I shouldn't be talking to any guys. My father could have stopped it, but he didn't.

Able to relate a concrete incident with father.

Therapist: What do you think about how your father behaved?

Encourages a cognitive appraisal of father.

Christine: He could have stopped Tom, but that's just my father, he never helped me. He didn't care. *(Pause)* …I think I had a dream about this…the other night.

Recognizes that father was not helpful and offers a dream indicating a positive alliance.

Therapist: Tell me about it.

Christine: My downstairs neighbor…you know, Wade…he's the one who is always coming up…he's disgusting…ugh, I can't stand him. My father is so nice to him. In the dream Wade came into our apartment, and he shot me in the stomach. It woke up the whole house, and my father came out of the bedroom…he saw I was shot. "Dad," I said, "get him out of the house." My father just stood there. "It's not so bad," he said. I started to cry and say, "Get help…." No one listened…no one helped. Suddenly, someone opened the door. A woman entered and called 911. I woke up…. It was 2:00 A.M. In my dream, my father didn't help me.

Relates dream about father's poor judgment, indifference, and neglect.

Therapist: It's true, he didn't seem to understand that you were injured and needed someone to help you. That's the way he's been much of your life. You have a good understanding of what kind of man your father is.

Agrees with Christine and offers praise.

Christine: That's the way he is. I guess no one helped him…his stepfather beat him and…he didn't get help, either. It's like we said, he can't do any better. That's it.

Realizes father's limitations and understands that he is not going to change.

Therapist: It's a painful realization, don't you think?

Empathic response.

Christine: Yes, I understand about him. It's funny, in the dream I tell him to get Wade out of the house. He *(father)* doesn't know what to do.... I can't count on him.

Therapist: You're right, but in your dream you knew what to do, you told your father to get Wade out of the house and to get help. In your dream you knew how to take charge and take care of yourself, even though you're wounded.

Combines support and exploration.

Christine: I did, I knew how badly I was hurt, even if my father didn't.

Therapist: This is the first dream you've told me in which you've taken charge and made sure you got the help you needed, and in your life, you did manage to get away from Tom, to get out of the car, even though you were wounded.

Continues to point out Christine's positive behavior. Indicates Christine's functional initiative in the therapy session.

Christine: That makes me feel better.

Therapist: Yes, in the dream your activity is reassuring. You know what to do, and if you can't do it alone, as in the dream, you create a helper like the woman in the dream.

Further exploration of the dream.

Christine: I do, she's the one who got help...called 911.

Therapist: Do you think she had anything to do with me?

Suggests a transference link.

Christine: I don't know...I couldn't make out her face, but she wore glasses...like yours.

Sees the connection.

Therapist: So the woman was me. In the dream, you took charge and I helped you, together we got help. Don't forget that you wrote the dream script, you're working out the trauma that you had with Tom, and now in your dream you're taking charge.

Christine: Yeah, and when I woke up, I wasn't so scared.

Indicates less traumatic anxiety.

Therapist: This time it was different, would you agree?

Christine: Yes, it was.

Therapist: I think you've made progress in a number of areas. Let's take some time to talk about it.

In this session, we can see Christine grappling with her parents' conflictual relationship, a mirror of the relationship she had with Tom. Working through the trauma of her relationship with Tom, the shootings, and her disappointment with her father leads to her dream. Although she is again shot, we can see more autonomy. In addition, the alliance and collaborative work with the therapist are part of the dream. These changes, coupled with her symptomatic relief, indicate that Christine may be ready for termination. The therapist sets the agenda for a review of Christine's progress, including what has been accomplished in her areas of disturbance. A reassessment is undertaken prior to termination.

Therapist: The major problem when you came to talk with me was your tremendous distress and inability to function in your usual way.

Begins the reassessment.

Christine: I'm not that way anymore. I thought I was falling apart and losing my mind, but now I feel better.

Therapist: What about the crying, the shaking, the anxiety and flashbacks?

Christine: No; sometimes I cry, but it's nothing like it was.

Acknowledges significant improvement.

Therapist: And your feelings about being Tom's murderer?

Continues review of Christine's areas of disturbance.

Christine: That's different. I know I didn't kill him. He was such a mess. He treated me so badly...I just took it. I loved him so much.

Therapist: Any thoughts?

Christine: It was...a mistake, I would never let anyone do that to me again. There's this guy at work, I told you about him, Larry. It's different with him...he's nice to me.

Indicates better object choice.

Therapist: You're feeling better and thinking better.

Points out improvement and enhances self-esteem.

Christine: Yeah, I'm moving with the company to their new offices and getting a raise. I spoke to my boss and asked for a raise.

Therapist: That's a good example of how you've been able to stand up for yourself.

Christine: I have been, and I'm going to get my own place...no more living with my parents.... Anyway, I want to be closer to work, so it makes sense.

Major shift in autonomy with separation from her parents.

Therapist: So you've made changes...done a lot of positive things, including how you think about yourself. It may be time to talk about ending therapy.

Formally raises the possibility of termination.

Christine: I've been thinking about that, but I was afraid to bring it up.

Therapist: How come?

Christine: I didn't know how you would take it.

Therapist: Were you concerned about my reaction; do you think you have to please me?

Addresses Christine's automatic thought, "If I act independently or assert myself, others will be disapproving and angry."

Christine: (*Somewhat hesitantly*) Well...I know, I probably don't
have to please you, but you've been so nice to me....

Expresses positive feelings for the therapist and recognition of her need to please.

Therapist: So you think that because you have positive feelings
for me, you can't risk asserting yourself, because you think
I would be unhappy or possibly angry with you?

Continues to explore patient's maladaptive behavior and automatic thinking.

Christine: I see what you mean, but it's not easy to change my way
of thinking.

States difficulty changing pattern of thinking.

Therapist: Remember when you went to the cemetery and you
thought I would be pleased? I wonder if you think you have
to please me or else I won't care about you.

Christine: Yeah, it was a good thing. You seemed to want me to
go, and even though I really knew Tom was dead, I couldn't
believe it.

Therapist: The need to please me is a concern of yours. The need
to please has been a large part of your life, and it's gotten you
into trouble with Tom. No matter how badly he treated you,
you kept trying to please him, without regard for your own
safety.

The session continued with further exploration of Christine's characteristic need to please and how it affects the termination process. Often, when
treatment is about to end, patients' characterological patterns and conflicts
reemerge in a relatively straightforward manner. Accordingly, an opportunity is presented to rework issues one more time.

Session 16

Christine: I saw Tom's brother at the train station yesterday. I was
scared, but it was all right. He said hello and asked how
I was.

Therapist: What did you expect to happen?

Explores.

Christine: I expected him to be angry, like in that dream I had a while ago, but... he wasn't. When I walked away from him, I felt better and was glad that I ran into him and it was okay. So he doesn't blame me for Tom's death.

Therapist: What about you? What's going on inside you?

Continues to explore.

Christine: I'm okay. Tom's gone, and when I think about the good times, I feel bad, but I know it's better for me without him.

Accepts Tom's death.

Therapist: You're right. It's interesting, you thought Tom's brother would give you a hard time, and last week you were afraid to bring up your concern about my reaction to your raising the issue of ending our work together.

Supports self-esteem and then links automatic thought about Tom's brother with the therapist.

Christine: I thought you wouldn't like it if I told you I wanted to stop. I thought you would get mad at me.

Reiterates automatic thought.

Therapist: What's the basis for your thought?

Asks for evidence.

Christine: I don't know, but you said it first, so you wouldn't have been mad at me. I thought you might be, so I didn't say anything.

Therapist: Could it be that you thought I might behave as Tom did when you wanted to end your relationship with him?

Transference link.

Christine: That's ridiculous... no, you didn't.

Therapist: I didn't, and neither did Tom's brother... so this is a thought that comes to your mind, an automatic way of thinking that you need to be mindful of.

Preparing patient for termination and the continued work on automatic thoughts after treatment ends.

Christine: So I still expect the worst, but not really.

Therapist: Last week we talked about ending treatment, so now we need to talk about saying goodbye to one another. How do you feel about stopping?

Returns to termination.

Christine: I feel ready, a lot has changed. Only...what if something happens...and I want to talk to you?

Indicates some hesitation.

Therapist: Would you call?

Explores.

Christine: Would I? Yes...so even when I leave, I can see you... you know, if something comes up?

Wants to know that therapist will be available.

Therapist: Sure, you can call me. I'd be glad to talk to you.

Reassures Christine of availability.

Christine: You would?

Expresses some doubt.

Therapist: Yes, I would; why wouldn't I? Can you think of a reason?

Reassures and explores.

Christine: Because I'm leaving.

Therapist: What do you feel about leaving me?

Shifts to Christine's feelings.

Christine: I feel upset.... I want to stop coming, but I like to talk to you. I know I still will have problems, but not like with Tom. I think I'm different now.

Expresses ambivalence about leaving but acknowledges change.

Therapist: How do you feel about saying goodbye to me?

Pursues Christine's feelings about the therapist.

Christine: Well... what I like is... it's that I'm learning from you... how I have habits... and how... not really wanting to... I've done things that got me into terrible trouble.... I won't do anything like that again... at least I hope not!

Avoids her feelings, but indicates that therapy has been a learning experience for her.

Therapist: You've learned a lot about yourself. Do you think you will continue the learning process on your own?

Acknowledges Christine's progress and suggests that she continue the work of therapy on her own.

Christine: I think so. I know how we discuss problems, and I can try to do the same thinking on my own.

Acknowledges that she can continue the work of therapy and has internalized the therapist function.

Therapist: Can you give me an example?

Takes a concrete approach.

Christine: We've talked about it. It's about moving out of my parents' apartment to be closer to work and be on my own. My father doesn't care if I move out, but my mother said she thinks I should wait till I get married to move out. She said that yesterday... no, the day before.

Therapist: What did you feel when she told you she thinks you should wait till you get married?

Explores.

Christine: I was annoyed. Here I am, planning to move, and I've said yes to my company that I will move with them, and now she starts to give me the guilt. I mean, I don't even have a boyfriend!

Therapist: You felt annoyed and then guilty about leaving your mother, is that it?

Clarification.

Christine: *(Nods yes.)*

Therapist: How did you think about what was occurring between you and your mother?

Asks patient to problem-solve.

Christine: I thought that moving out is a good thing for me. It makes sense. I'll be close to work and I want to be on my own. My mother wants me to be around because she likes the company. But she won't die if I leave. *(Starts to laugh)* I can't believe I said that.

Shows ability to solve problems and diminished automatic thinking.

Therapist: But that's your struggle, you feel you have matured and can make a positive change in your life, but at the same time you're afraid that if you go off on your own, there'll be terrible consequences.

Addresses Christine's statement about mother's death with a link to the traumatic event with Tom.

Christine: Yes, but that's not true. My mother won't die if I leave. It's not like with Tom.

Demonstrates a shift in thinking.

Therapist: And she won't shoot you either. You'll both work it out, even though you think differently.

Uses humor and reassurance.

Christine: Yes, that's the truth. We get along pretty well.

Therapist: Getting back to us...I think you were concerned that I, like your mother, want you to stay, and that even getting in touch with me again would be complicated because of it. Does that make sense?

Connects termination with leaving mother (transference link).

Christine: Oh, it's that same thing, I expected that you would be angry at me for leaving.

Therapist: Right, like Tom was and your mother. But that doesn't mean you can't do what makes sense for you.

Christine: Yes, I know.

Therapist: How do you feel now about saying goodbye to me? Earlier you spoke about your concerns about saying goodbye, but do you have any other feelings about our ending our work together?

Asks for other feelings about termination which have only been expressed as fears.

Christine: You helped me a lot. I feel sad about saying goodbye. I really like talking to you, and I looked forward to seeing you every week. Now I don't need to see you, and it's okay.

Therapist: I also feel sad about saying goodbye to you. I've enjoyed our work together.

Termination with Christine was relatively uncomplicated. Although the therapist introduced the subject, the patient acknowledged that she had thought about ending treatment. In fact, work on termination presented an opportunity for a corrective emotional experience, since the patient expected the therapist to react negatively to her desire to end treatment. She was surprised when the therapist raised the subject, and understood that her habitual way of thinking did not have a basis in reality.

Case 3: Expressive-Supportive Psychotherapy— Sarah's Choice

In the midphase of treatment, Sarah was able to work through issues related to pathological mourning, particularly as it related to her relationship with her mother. As a result, she felt less guilty about choosing to separate from her mother during the selection process in the concentration camp. Her habit of opposing others, judging them harshly, and attributing malicious motives to them was identified as partially fueled by her experience in the concentration camp and no longer adaptive. Her automatic negative thoughts, although not absent, have yielded to the reality of the present. During the midphase, Sarah's view of her older son's upcoming marriage as a loss to be endured yielded to a somewhat more positive one, enabling her to participate in social functions planned by her future daughter-in-law's family. She was also successful at finding a job.

Session 17

> Sarah: *(Appears distressed and has an edge in her voice)* I'm very busy at work; I had to leave in the middle of something to come here.

Suggests some reluctance about coming to the session.

> Therapist: What are you feeling now?

Recognizes Sarah's reluctance and begins to explore.

> Sarah: ...Harried, it's not your fault.... I wanted to finish my work before I left the office. I like to be effective, and don't like rushing off before I'm done.

Indicates she would have preferred to remain at work. May be an allusion to ending treatment.

> Therapist: Yes, I can see that; how do you feel about hurrying here when you also wanted to remain at work?

Clarifies Sarah's conflict.

> Sarah: Well, to be late, or not to come at all, I wouldn't do that...I have been thinking that I'm ready to put an end to our meetings.

Explains that her conflict is based on her wish to end treatment.

> Therapist: Do you think feeling harried is related to your thought of ending treatment?

Explores connection of Sarah's wish to end therapy and feeling harried.

> Sarah: I think it is. I foresee that you will not want me to go and will get angry at me for wanting to stop.

Agrees and elaborates on the association of feeling harried and ending treatment.

Therapist: So this harried feeling is also a response to my anticipated anger (*Sarah nods in agreement*). What makes you think
I will be angry or irritated if you wish to leave treatment?

Clarifies and explores.

Sarah: I've been thinking about stopping for the last few days.
Manners, that's important, remember I'm European. What
would be good manners? This has been a sweet acquaintance, and I don't want to spoil it.

Indicates a concern about therapist's reaction to her wish to stop.

Therapist: "A sweet acquaintance"...yes, it has been that, but
let's examine your thought that I'll be angry if you stop treatment.

*Picks up on Sarah's positive statement about therapist and then explores possi-
ble cognitive distortion.*

Sarah: I don't know, I always used to watch for slights or disre-
gards, or grudges. I don't want you to hold a grudge when
I leave. I've been working all my life so that no one could become too important, and I have succeeded, except with my
sons and now with you.

Admits that therapist has become important to her.

Therapist: When you think about stopping treatment, you worry
about what I'll think about you, because I've become important in your life.

Clarifies.

Sarah: Yes, that's true, I want to leave here and I want you to agree
with me and still care about me.

Expresses need for therapist's approval of her wish to leave.

Therapist: Saying goodbye won't change my positive feelings for
you...saying goodbye won't change our sweet acquaintance. But why don't we take a little time today to see how
things are in your life now. Does that make sense to you?

*Reassures Sarah that therapist's positive feeling for her will persist and suggests
a more leisurely goodbye—a different and corrective experience.*

> Sarah: I suppose so. I'm successful at work now. You know, it's not
> like it was on my other job. They appreciate me... and I feel
> flattered when they ask my opinion on business matters.

> Therapist: And your regard for yourself.... You feel worthy now?

Therapist's statement is in the form of a question to see of there is agreement.

> Sarah: It's better, yes. I like this job. I'm not just doing clerical work.
> Whatever goes out, the orders, all the correspondence related
> to the orders, I check to see if it's feasible for us to do the work.

> Therapist: And with Martin, your boss?

> Sarah: He likes me.

> Therapist: So work is much better. And how are things going with
> Ernest?

> Sarah: Well, with Ernest it's never going to be perfect, but we're
> getting along okay now. I used to think I got my position
> from my husband, from hanging onto his coattails. How he
> treated me made me feel I was more or less important. I'm
> not angry at him so much of the time. When I talk to Ernest,
> I know I'm not talking to an enemy. He cares about me, but
> he's European and he expects me to be a certain way....

The session continued with the patient talking about her relationship
with her husband, which is much improved. She feels close to her son, accepts his marriage, and looks forward to a positive relationship with his wife
and in-laws. Sarah has more positive thoughts and feelings toward her mother
and can tolerate her profound sadness over her losses. Therapist and patient
agreed to meet two more times and then end treatment.

Session 18

> Sarah: Ernest has been difficult. I don't know what to do with
> him. He's been so critical. Steven (*her son*) brought me flow-
> ers on Friday. I was so happy... I was thinking maybe I can
> visit Steven's future in-laws. But then Ernest didn't like it
> that Steven brought me flowers.

*Presents conflict with husband. Conflicts as well as new information will often
emerge during the termination process. These need not alter the termination
schedule if the patient's progress and adaptation are maintained.*

Therapist: How did that make you feel?

Explores feeling.

Sarah: I was angry. I was all set to walk out, then I thought, "You can never let me be happy...but I'm not going to get into a war about this." I didn't walk out; I put the flowers on the table and we had dinner.

Describes adaptive behavior.

Therapist: That's a big change for you. You knew you were angry, considered your choices, didn't go to war, and allowed yourself to enjoy the evening with your family. Did you eventually talk with Ernest when the two of you were alone?

Clarifies, praises, and explores.

Sarah: Yes, I told him he turns things negative. I was happy about the flowers, and he didn't like it. He got jealous.

Therapist: How did you resolve it?

Solution-focused question.

Sarah: Well, Ernest backed down. When I talk strongly to him, he responds. He wasn't really mad, he was jealous of my relationship with Steven (*able to differentiate affect and can respond differentially*). My relationship with Steven is really nice. We talk together and get along well. He's proud of me.

Therapist: And you, how do you feel about yourself?

Sarah: I feel better, good. You are part of it...it's different.... We talk, and you can take my anger and still like me.

Indicates improved self-esteem and a positive view of the patient-therapist relationship.

Therapist: I do like you. Your anger, well, that's just one way you respond to me sometimes, and we've learned a lot from that, don't you think?

Expresses positive feelings for Sarah and indicates that examining Sarah's anger was a useful learning experience.

Sarah: I know, but somehow it's what stands out. I'll have more of a family now that Steven is getting married, and it's good for Isaac (her younger son). I don't want to be like vinegar. At first it was hard for me to manage it all. I never had anyone walk me through anything...my marriage, or having children.... Ernest had no family. It means a lot to have a family.

Agrees that the therapist has provided a learning experience.

Therapist: So we've been doing a walk-through. In life, ordinarily, anger doesn't end relationships—it didn't end ours, and it wasn't your anger that caused the destruction of your family. Sometimes you forget, but being assertive the way you were then and can be now, with some tact, makes sense, and generally there are no consequences of significance.

Clarifies Sarah's view of anger and assertiveness.

Sarah: I can remember how it was with my father. On Saturdays, I went walking with him.

Brings up a new memory, but based on the walking-through with the therapist.

Therapist: How was your father with you?

Explores.

Sarah: He liked me and thought I was someone to be proud of. I think he was proud of me. He didn't mind to have platonic romances with other women.

Indicates father's pride in her and interest in other women.

Therapist: Oh, with who?

Sarah: He used to flirt with the neighbor's wife. She wasn't a knockout, but he thought he was a Don Juan. He enjoyed looking at women.

Therapist: And with you?

Focuses on possible flirtation between Sarah and her father.

Sarah: On one Saturday when I was walking with my father, I took his arm. (*Smiling*) I said, "Let's play adults." We walked like honeymooners.... I was maybe 10. I wish we'd had more time together.

Describes her flirtation with her father and her longing for more time with him.

Therapist: Last week we agreed that we would have two more sessions and then stop treatment. Now you're talking about wishing for more time with your father. Do you think this has something to do with me?

Links wish for more time with father to termination.

Sarah: When I first came to see you, I was in a terrible mood, was facing a wedding and dealing with a new family. It's better now...I really don't have to come...I'm not so emotionally constipated anymore. Don't get me wrong, I can still be ice, but it's nice to talk to you.

Indicates that she wants to end treatment.

Therapist: You like to talk to me, but clearly you have mixed feelings about stopping...saying goodbye to me.

Confronts Sarah's mixed feelings.

Sarah: That's true. I used to feel that I was never important enough...that I got leftovers. Now I know it's not true. I was close to my father, and even though I wish my mother was warmer toward me, she cared about me.

Connects her positive feelings toward therapist with father and mother.

Therapist: What you're saying is very important. Your perception of your mother and father is different now. You can feel tenderness toward them while at the same time acknowledging what a terrible loss you sustained. A few moments ago I asked how you felt about saying goodbye to me. How do you feel?

Empathically clarifies and then focuses on Sarah's feelings about saying goodbye to the therapist.

Sarah: How do I feel? Yesterday was the sixth day that I didn't see you, and I was thinking that I don't have to come anymore, but I also realized that the days between somehow don't exist for me.

Therapist: And...?

Sarah: It makes me look forward to our times together.

Expresses longing for therapist.

Therapist: Do you notice you're sort of talking about your feelings toward me, but not directly about saying goodbye?

Confronts Sarah's partial declaration of feeling for therapist.

Sarah: Well, it's hard. I'm going to miss seeing you.

Therapist: And the feeling?

Recognizes Sarah's difficulty being direct with her feelings toward therapist.

Sarah: I feel good with you, you understand. It makes me feel sad.
Anyway, Ernest wants me to stop.

Avoids feeling.

Therapist: Again you are moving away from the sadness.

Confronts Sarah's defensive avoidance.

Sarah: Thinking about this makes me weepy. I don't want to be
like that. I've had enough sadness in my life.

Connects difficulty with her sad feelings to her previous losses.

Therapist: You're right, but it's important for us to know what you
are feeling and for you to allow yourself to have these feelings. You've lost so many people in your life. This time saying goodbye is not so final.

Clarifies and underlines importance of Sarah's feelings about leaving therapist.

The session began with Sarah expressing angry feelings toward her husband but indicating that she was able to recognize her feelings and deal with
them in an appropriate and adaptive manner. After some clarifying and confrontation of Sarah's defensiveness, she was able to reveal her positive feelings for the therapist, indicating that with the therapist she had experienced
"a walk-through," or rehearsal, of important life events. This experience and
her feelings for the therapist evoked a pleasant memory of taking walks with

her father and the wish that she had had more time with him. An important memory occurring after exploration of the patient-therapist relationship is generally indicative of a correct approach or intervention. The session concluded with more work on Sarah's feelings about leaving treatment and their connection to previous losses. The work of termination in patients who have suffered significant loss invariably includes linking the loss of the therapist with other important losses in the patient's life.

Session 19

> Sarah: I was thinking about my mother. You remember, I told you I wanted to stay with the older girls in the selection. Obedience counted in my family, but I always wanted to get away with it. My mother wanted me to stay with her, but I went off with the older girls. My mother...she should have held on to me.

The adaptive context is again loss. This has been a repeated theme throughout treatment and is evoked and heightened by the termination process.

> Therapist: What meaning does that have for us? We've been talking about ending treatment and saying goodbye, and today is our last session.

Links loss of mother with loss of therapist.

> Sarah: I want to go now....

Defensive avoidance.

> Therapist: But you wished your mother would have held on to you.... Is it the same with me?

Confronts defensive avoidance.

> Sarah: I don't know...yes.... It's like I'm going to be alone again. I know I can stand up for myself, but it's terrible to be alone.

Expresses feelings of loneliness.

> Therapist: Tell me.

Explores.

Sarah: I was only a child...worthless...powerless to have my wishes considered. Whatever happened had nothing to do with me. They were Gods...I was powerless.

Expresses her powerlessness in the concentration camp setting, but appears to understand what she experienced as a child.

Therapist: Is that the way it is here with us?

Explores therapeutic relationship.

Sarah: *(Long pause)* In a way.... I want to go, but I want you to hold on to me.

Expresses conflict about saying goodbye to therapist, which may be related to letting go of mother.

Therapist: And how would that be if I said no, stay with me?

Asks for fantasy.

Sarah: *(Laughing)* I would feel you care about me...that I am important, not just a patient.

Reveals Sarah's wish for a special relationship with therapist. It is likely also an expression of the transference with a connection to her mother. Because this is the end of therapy, the therapist chooses to emphasize the real relationship.

Therapist: I do care about you and really like being with you. But we both know it's time to say goodbye.

Expresses genuine positive feelings for Sarah and concurs in her wish to leave treatment and be autonomous. This constitutes a corrective emotional experience, given that the therapist is not pressing her to remain, the way her mother did.

Sarah: I know.

Therapist: We've seen how much you've improved. Your wish to end treatment makes sense, as did your wish to be independent when you were 13. Now you're a woman with resources, and you have a family that is enlarging. Back then, you were still a child going to a death camp.

Evidence-based praise with emphasis on the difference between her past and current life.

Sarah: I have to handle my life.

Therapist: It's time to say goodbye. It's been a pleasure to have had the opportunity to work with you these past months. And you know where to find me if the need arises.

A genuine expression of feelings about working with the patient emphasizes the real relationship and promotes a positive alliance that lives on after treatment ends. Reminding patients of the therapist's availability after termination again helps maintain a positive alliance and is reassuring to the patient.

Sarah began the session with thoughts about the loss of her mother, which was linked to terminating with the therapist (interpretation in the triangle of person). Further exploration of the patient-therapist relationship was undertaken, which led to a corrective emotional experience vis-à-vis ending without a struggle. Sarah was able to say goodbye to the therapist without being pressured to remain in treatment. It goes without saying that the therapist also sustains a loss at termination, and it is always necessary for the therapist to be mindful of his or her own personal experiences with loss that may affect the work of termination. Such an awareness helps the therapist understand what the patient is experiencing and diminishes negative countertransference reactions.

Case 4: Expressive Psychotherapy—
The Man Who Never Said Goodbye

Early losses of the important people in Mark's life made termination a complicated and emotionally wrenching process for him. His mother and father had died before he was 5 years old, and he lost his aunt and uncle during the next several years. The loss of a significant person can come alive in the therapeutic relationship and enable the patient to explore sadness, loss, attachment, anger, and other feelings directly within the patient-therapist relationship. In this treatment, the termination process involved mourning the loss of the therapist. The reality of ending treatment affords the patient the opportunity to rework earlier losses by linking the loss of the therapist to the people lost in childhood. The issue of termination was raised by both patient and therapist, since this treatment was entered into as brief therapy of 30 sessions.

These processes will be illustrated using excerpts from the last four sessions.

Session 27

Mark: I was thinking about all the work I do, getting information for everyone at work. I don't seem to get credit for what I do. It gets me more and more angry. Actually, I felt so angry that I nearly started yelling at people at work.

The adaptive context appears to be that Mark works hard and perceives himself as unappreciated.

Therapist: So you've been angry about not being recognized and appreciated at work, but it sounds like this anger may be an overreaction. Is something else going on? Maybe the recognition and appreciation you seek at work is also something you want from me and other important people in your life.

Links Mark's anger with patient-therapist relationship.

Mark: I'm feeling down, but also involved... knowing I'm coming to see you... someone who listens to me... not like the people at work.

Denies anger toward therapist and acknowledges feeling downhearted.

Therapist: Perhaps part of your reaction is related to the fact that we have to say goodbye to one another.

Links Mark's feeling down with termination.

Mark: Yes, that's why I'm feeling down. What am I going to do?

Acknowledges feeling, but moves to helpless position.

Therapist: Before we jump to what you're going to do, let's try to see what you're feeling and experiencing about saying goodbye to me.

Holds patient to feelings about ending.

Mark: I'm going to be depressed and not able to make up for the loss. I'm very angry with you. We are achieving things together *(slams hand on table)*, and now we're stopping and you won't be with me. This always happens to me.

Able to be direct with therapist.

Therapist: It's clear that a lot of your anger is toward me, not just toward the people at work.

Addresses displacement of anger.

Mark: The closer I get to terminating with you, the more angry I get with people at work.

Confirmation of interpretation of defense.

Therapist: You shift your anger to people at work, but you're really angry with me. Let's stay with your anger toward me.

Holds Mark to anger in patient-therapist relationship.

Mark: I'm just so angry that it's going to be over, I want to continue with you. I begin to wonder if you care about me, and I get more upset and angry.

Therapist: So there is a lot of anger in you toward me.

Mark: Yes, why can't we continue? You don't have to stop. I need to keep seeing you. I'll be lost *(looks visibly sad)*.

A new affect is emerging.

Therapist: I wonder if it's all anger, because now you look sad and there are tears in your eyes. We know you ward off other deeper feelings with anger. What else are you feeling?

Asks for other feelings related to nonverbal communication.

Mark: I'm feeling very sad. When I'm with you it's like being in a timeless universe, with a big bubble around us. When I leave, that's it ... a real loss.

Acknowledges sadness.

Therapist: You're saying you won't carry any of our work together with you after therapy is over?

Asks for Mark to recognize what he has internalized as a result of their collaborative effort.

Mark: As we get to the end, it's starting to disappear...I'm losing you. It's like I have no strength. I'm impotent without you.

Regresses to feeling that without therapist, he is helpless.

> Therapist: What about all of our work together?—you will take
> that with you.

The therapist goes on to explain that the patient has made a major contribution to the success of therapy and that the process of working through
conflicts and problems can continue after therapy is over. Acknowledging
the patient's work in treatment helps to decrease patient passivity and promote more active mastery for the patient over the termination process. In addition, the therapist explains that the patient will take with him all of the
accomplishments of their work together, helping to further the patient's
identification with the therapist. Mark continues to talk about his feelings
about the loss of the therapist, and the therapist links these feelings to Mark's
previous losses.

Session 28

> Mark: Sue got very angry with me this weekend. We went to
> Washington to visit her brother. I was preoccupied and
> uninvolved...I guess mostly because of leaving therapy
> with you. The other issue on my mind was work—I'm not
> making enough progress. Then I got upset with my daugh-
> ter...shook her...and then, going home from Washington,
> when we stopped to eat, I was irritable with Sue and the
> kids. I just felt frustrated.

The adaptive context continues to be termination of therapy.

> Therapist: Let's look at this. We are coming to the end of therapy,
> and all of a sudden you are reverting back to becoming either
> irritable or uninvolved.

*Points out return of past maladaptive behavior. During the termination process,
symptoms often return which may constitute a plea from the patient to be allowed to continue therapy.*

> Mark: Yes, it's hard to stop treatment. I'm getting angry...I was
> doing so well, and now...

> Therapist: You're angry about stopping treatment...angry with
> me and displacing it onto Sue and the kids. You either be-
> come irritable and impulsive or withdrawn and passive.

Links anger with termination.

Mark: Well, I still need treatment. This shows that I do.

Therapist: But you leave out your prior progress. You were doing well, and then, as we start to say goodbye to each other, you start to get worse. So having difficulty now is directly tied to your feelings about me and our stopping treatment.

Reminds patient of his improvement and connects current difficulties with termination.

Mark: Coming here today, I was thinking I don't know what to say. Then I saw you and I felt sad.

Therapist: As we've seen many times, underneath your anger is a lot of sadness. Let's look at your sadness in relation to me.

Mark: The sadness is a longing. I can't seem to get it together.

Therapist: Our saying goodbye leads you to feel sad and long for me.

Clarifies.

Mark: I think the strength I've been feeling within myself comes from you. If I lose you, I'll fall apart.

Regression and yearning.

Therapist: You're dismissing all you've done and the progress you've made…your strengths and accomplishments.

Focuses on Mark's strengths instead of his regressive behavior.

Mark: I saw how strong my rage was and how my rage is a cover for so much sadness in me.

Insight.

Therapist: You said how sad you are about losing me, and then we saw how you got angry with Sue and the kids.

Mark: I guess it reminds me of all the losses that I've had.

Links prior losses to termination.

Therapist: I don't think it's a guess. We know that you've had terrible losses in your life, and it's been hard for you to go back and talk about the losses and the sad feelings. It's much harder for you than the angry feelings.

Explanation of complicated layers of feelings.

Mark: Yes, longing and loss is very hard for me. I feel Sue is abusing me by demanding that I function when I feel so bad... but I feel so sad, it's so deep.

Feelings toward Sue may be an allusion to the therapist.

Therapist: So the losses that you've had come back to haunt you.

Ignores Mark's feelings of abuse and continues to connect termination with past losses.

Mark: Yes, I keep thinking that my center is filled with sadness... I can't separate myself from my past. I'm trying to understand what happened to me, but at the same time I have to function in the present. I can't preoccupy myself with the past.

Therapist: That's true, but here with me we can look at all these feelings.

Agrees with the importance of Mark's functioning in the present, but continues to explore feelings.

Mark: I feel like you're dying.

Therapist: So I'm dying in your life.

Mark: Yes, like my mother and father, but now I feel it with you. If you leave my life, I'm going to feel diminished. How will I accomplish things? I keep going back to my earlier life... seeing frailties in my mother, father, brother. They viewed me as a burden.

Links termination with loss of mother and father.

Therapist: You see their frailties and think that they viewed you as a burden. How about me...do you think I view you as a burden, and that's why therapy is ending?

Connects parents and therapist.

> Mark: No, but I do feel that if you really cared about me, you wouldn't stop the therapy. It's too short. I need more time. I feel very strongly about you, and I like to think you have some kind of feeling for me.... I think you do, but I depend on you...I need you.

Continues to express need for therapist.

> Therapist: I know it's hard for you. Each step is difficult, and it's hard for you to take off and be independent. But you have made a great deal of progress. You said you'd like to think I have feelings for you. I do. I've enjoyed working with you. Our work together has been very important to me.

Expresses empathy and positive feelings, indicating that Mark was not a burden.

> Mark: That's important for me to hear. It means a lot to me to feel that you care about me.

> The patient then goes on to speak of his growing closeness to his wife and children and his greater productivity at work.

In this session, the patient brought up his yearning for the therapist and his feeling that there is a well of sadness at his center. Anger was interpreted as a defense against Mark's sadness and his wish to be cared for by the therapist. These feelings were linked to the early loss of his parents. The therapist then expressed positive feelings for the patient, indicating that there was pleasure in working together. This direct expression of feeling by the therapist was positively received by Mark. A direct statement like this may seem like a departure from expressive therapy; however, it is not unusual for the therapist in integrated therapy containing interpersonal elements to directly express feelings to the patient. Self-revelation is appropriate, provided it is in the service of the patient and not the therapist.

The termination in Mark's therapy is filled with many feelings, yearning, and regressive wishes. These inevitably lead to therapist countertransference feelings. Most people have difficulty with separation and loss, and therapists are no exception. It is important for therapists to monitor their feelings to avoid side-stepping these difficult issues. At times in this session, the therapist chose to link Mark's feelings toward the therapist with figures from the past. The therapist always has to make choices and at times will make mistakes. In this session, the patient preferred to stay in the present, in effect helping to keep therapy on course.

Session 29

> Mark: This is our next-to-the-last session.

Adaptive context continues to be termination.

> Therapist: That's right. How do you feel about it?

> Mark: I feel better since we've been talking about it some.

Exploring termination appears to be helpful.

> Therapist: So we need to talk about it a lot more, not just some.

> Mark: After the last session, I realized I felt some tension. I felt losing you as a therapist was making it difficult for me to progress. Then I remembered that during a previous session, you said, "People often continue to progress after therapy is over." I also felt that just in acknowledging our stopping I feel better, but I still don't feel really good.

Able to use information conveyed by therapist.

> Therapist: So on the positive side, what you learned from our work together was helpful and made you feel better, but there's still tension centered around our stopping.

A supportive clarification is offered, followed by an invitation to continue exploring termination.

> Mark: The conflict was about stopping, but the difference here with you is that for the first time in my life, I'm getting to talk about the loss of a significant figure in my life with the actual person. Even in my long-term therapy, I never talked about leaving. I abruptly stopped the therapy.

Recognizes significance of this experience with the therapist, which is a working-through of the powerful feelings and conflicts related to loss of parents and other important people in his life, which he was unable to do as a child and with past therapist (corrective emotional experience).

> Therapist: So talking with me about saying goodbye is a first.

Mark: Yes, this is different, and I feel like I really have you. I couldn't do this with the other therapist, I just left.

Suggests an internalization of therapist function. Realizes that talking directly to the therapist about loss has helped.

Therapist: So you never talked to him about stopping.

Continues exploration.

Mark: He said I shouldn't stop, but I couldn't continue, because I started a new job. I never went back.

Rationalizes behavior with past therapist.

Therapist: So you never gave yourself a chance to talk about your feelings toward him at the end, about losing him.

Mark: Right.

Therapist: And we know you didn't get a chance to talk about your loss of your mother or father.

Utilizes the triangle of the person to link loss of parents with previous therapist and current therapist.

Mark: My grandfather, too. It still astounds me that no one thought he was significant in my life. They didn't even tell me he died until much later. This was a man who meant something to me. He was an exceptionally nice person who was gentle with me. He was just very nice. As I talk about my fond feelings for him, I realize I have similar feelings for you. I guess this is the problem... I felt better last week when I felt I could talk about this, and now when I talk more about my feelings toward you... it's hard to do.

Extends the sphere of loss to grandfather and links grandfather with therapist. Adopts therapist's mode of functioning (analyzing).

Therapist: I know it's hard for you, but it's important that we continue to examine your feelings toward me.

Empathizes and holds patient to continued work on ending.

Mark: I don't know. At some point yesterday, I felt I had a new outlook. I said to myself that I've been more troubled than

I realize. The issue is for me to acknowledge my feelings toward you. At the moment of loss it's very painful...I want to continue so my feelings can keep building up and go on forever. Now I realize that something is going to change here. It's too painful to deal with...that makes you incredibly important, but maybe you can just be someone I had a good and positive experience with. The problem, in part, was that I never conveyed to people I lost how important they were to me.

This statement reflects Mark's recognition of the therapist as a real person with whom he had a positive relationship. He is direct about his positive feelings toward therapist.

Therapist: I think you have conveyed to me how important I am to you and that I am someone you had a good and positive experience with.

Underlines Mark's positive statements.

Mark: Yes, but it's still painful to acknowledge how important you are to me.

Therapist: And the pain...what's that like?

Further exploration.

Mark: Like butterflies in my stomach. It makes me feel weak.

Therapist: Butterflies in your stomach...that sounds like anxiety, but as you talk there is a pervasive feeling of sadness that comes across too. Is that right?

Clarifies anxiety and interprets it as a reaction of underlying sadness (triangle of conflict).

Mark: Well, there is the fear that I can't function when I stop seeing you.

Avoids sadness in a regressive manner.

Therapist: So there is anxiety about the future and not being able to function without me. And the sadness?

Clarifies and continues to focus on sadness.

> Mark: You won't be a reality in my life, and I'll be spending time conjuring up the reality of you... trying to remember.

Grappling with difficulty incorporating therapist into his life.

> ·Therapist: So you're going to try to remember me. We've worked together, you've accomplished a lot... and what you've accomplished should stay with you.

Praises and indicates that patient has incorporated functions of therapist.

> Mark: I hope so, but the loss makes everything else unreal. It keeps me stuck in the same place. I need another way of looking at this.

Asks for reframing.

> Therapist: The way to look at this is to remember that your life has changed. You know what you feel, and you now use adaptive ways of coping with your loving and angry feelings. Your relationships with Sue and the children are quite good and the same is true for work. It sounds as if without me everything disappears—all your gains—when you stop seeing me, but you will take these with you. You make it sound as if you had nothing to do with all the changes you've made.

Reminds Mark of real progress.

> Mark: That's the way I feel.

> Therapist: I understand, but then you're giving me all the credit for your gains here. It's just not the case. You're leaving yourself out... all of your accomplishments... all of your hard work, have you forgotten that?

Reframes as a memory problem.

> Mark: No, I haven't forgotten! But the overriding reality is that this is not going to continue... it's over. You won't exist for me anymore.

Returns to negative view by negating therapist's existence as he did with other key people in his life.

> Therapist: So we have to say goodbye, but you make it sound as if I'm going to be dead in your life. In fact, you almost used those words.

Points out that Mark equates termination with death.

>   Mark: Well you will drift away as time goes on...further away...I can picture it. It's like the picture in the Sistine Chapel by Michelangelo. Adam and God drifting apart. This describes the world better than anything else...at least to me.

Idealizes therapist and recognizes the imminence of separation.

>   Therapist: You're right, we do have to say goodbye.

>   Mark: Even to talk about the grief is a tremendous gain for me. I want to reach out to you...like Michelangelo's Adam and God. I'm putting it in reverse. No sooner do they touch, then they drift apart...they're being swept away.

Recognizes positive experience of talking about separation.

>   Therapist: You feel we've touched and now we are going to drift apart?

Clarifies.

>   Mark: Yeah, even though I haven't had a chance to fully know you, something good has happened here, but I need more time to make it real. It's not real enough...that's what I'm afraid of. At the same time, I want to get closer to my kids. They don't get enough of me. They are very fond of me, and I really care about them.

Shifts to children.

>   Therapist: You really have warm, positive feelings for your kids.

Decides to focus on patient's feelings toward his children rather than comment on Mark's wish for more time, because these were positive and adaptive.

>   Mark: All my problems were problems for my kids. As I perform better, I'll be able to set up a more secure environment for my children. You seem to be smiling.

Reveals wish to be more active and productive.

>   Therapist: Yes, I am. Do you have some thoughts about my smiling?

>   Mark: I think that you thought there was something good in me for feeling that way...that what I was saying touched you.

Understands that therapist admires him.

> Therapist: It did. You're right, your concern and love for your children touch me very much.

Acknowledges feelings.

> Mark: There is so much feeling in me that is starting to emerge. You can't imagine how much this has meant to me.

The session began with Mark indicating that talking about termination has been helpful. Mark's remembering the therapist's saying that people continue to progress after therapy ends reflects Mark's incorporation of what he has learned from the therapist. A corrective emotional experience takes place in Mark's life, because this is the first time he has been able to say goodbye to the person he will lose. He is able to experience his feelings toward the therapist, a benign figure in the present—feelings that were formerly intolerable and unbearable. As this occurs, he is able to develop some mastery over the experience of loss. Mark is able to see the therapist as both important to him and a real person. The therapist linked termination with Mark's loss of his parents, an interpretation utilizing the triangle of the person. Mark was able to extend this interpretation to his grandfather, indicating that he has been able to internalize the therapist functions.

At the same time, he continued to exhibit regressive behavior, stating that he might be unable to function when treatment stops. Regressive behavior is not unusual during the termination process, especially when a person has suffered from multiple losses. He also expressed anxiety, sadness, and grief, which the therapist continued to explore. Mark's God/Adam metaphor reveals idealization of the therapist with recognition that they have touched one another's lives but must inevitably drift apart. It is an acceptance of the reality of ending.

Session 30

> Mark: Last session!

> Therapist: That's right.

> Mark: I have an image of myself standing by the door overcome with emotion...crying. I say if this is the way I feel, how can I function? I know I like to feel my feelings. Is there something wrong with me?

Begins with a regressive fantasy.

Therapist: That you have feelings?

Mark: It makes me feel that I'm weak.

Continues with theme of regression.

Therapist: The fact that you have strong feelings is important. It's curious that you take this as a sign of weakness. This may go back to the time when you had trouble handling your feelings. Now it's different. You have them and can handle them.

Reframes regression and points out Mark's ability to cope, thereby discouraging regression.

Mark: Yeah. I want a world where I can have feelings, but it's a cold place. It doesn't look too kindly on my having them.

Therapist: That's exactly what we've been working on. Your feelings are important and critical. How you show them is another story, as you know. When you were leaving here last time, you said something very important.

Mark: What I remember saying is, "You can't imagine how much this has meant to me."

Reflects Mark's investment in the work of therapy.

Therapist: So there are a lot of very deep feelings within you toward me.

Continues to emphasize how Mark feels.

Mark: I'm feeling sad about leaving you.

Responds in a more mature rather than a regressive manner.

Therapist: So in terms of our saying goodbye to one another, you've told me about the sadness and about the good feelings toward me and how this is the first time you've been able to say goodbye to someone who is important to you.

Emphasizes the positive aspects of termination.

Mark: It's real important. You're the first person I could say goodbye to who is around and important to me (*sighs*). I want to
say goodbye again.

Agrees with therapist.

Therapist: And what are you feeling now?

Mark: This has been a wonderful experience for me. It would have
been better if it was longer, but it's remarkable. So much of
this had to do with you... you're so suited to my needs.

Expresses appreciation of therapist's qualities.

Therapist: I appreciate your positive feelings toward me, but a lot
of your progress had to do with you. You worked hard and
made a big difference.

Expresses appreciation and praises patient for his hard work.

Mark: In other words, I felt this was important and I worked
hard.

Therapist: Yes, you made a major effort and we did it together.

Mark: You're giving a gift to me that I want to continue to
use... to give myself a better life... both internally for myself
and to my family. I want to give more love to Sue and to my
children. I have to work on these. I have to value my feelings
and to recognize them.

The final session illustrates that Mark came to terms about separation
and loss. He was able to value his work in treatment as a collaborative effort.
As Mark worked through saying goodbye to the therapist, he was able to
shift his focus to his wife and children. He turned to the reality of his life situation and away from the therapist, which is appropriate.

Conclusions

In the termination phase of psychotherapy, the emphasis is on saying goodbye. Three of the four patients presented in this chapter went through the
termination process in their own characteristic way. Christine still had concerns about pleasing others and did not initiate the termination process even
though she thought about ending treatment. Sarah signaled her wish to end

treatment by coming late to a session; rather than being direct and clear, she expected the therapist to know what she was thinking, just as she had expected this of her husband. Mark's termination reflected his inability to recognize himself as a strong individual, attributing his improvement entirely to the therapist. Although Lucy stated that she was ready to end treatment and was pleased about the changes in her functioning and mood, the therapist suggested continuation of treatment, primarily for medication maintenance.

The three patients who terminated continued to work through their interpersonal problems within the framework of ending treatment with the therapist. With each patient, the therapist identified the patient's characteristic way of coping with termination, making connections between the patient's behavior with the therapist and the patient's behavior with other important people in his or her life. In addition, patients such as Sarah and Mark had a chance to rework significant losses in the here-and-now of the patient-therapist relationship and come to a better understanding and resolution of these losses.

CHAPTER

10

Research in Brief Psychotherapy

In the past 15 to 20 years, psychotherapy research has flourished, and its methods have become more sophisticated. For all practical purposes, most researchers in psychotherapy have used brief psychotherapy as the model for study. Research on long-term therapy, with the possible exception of process studies, is too costly and impractical to be used on an ongoing basis. Although our focus in this chapter is outcome research, we also discuss relevant process research directly connected to outcome.

Outcome research can examine either ultimate outcome or immediate outcome. *Ultimate outcome* refers to improvement measured at termination and/or at follow-up some time later. *Immediate outcome* refers to change occurring within a smaller time frame, such as a session or a segment of a session. Generally, measurement of such aspects as symptoms, functioning, well-being, interpersonal behavior, and personality dimensions is used to determine outcome. Process measurements concern everything that can be observed to occur between patient and therapist on a moment-to-moment basis. The distinction between outcome research—particularly immediate-outcome research—and process research is somewhat blurred. For example, when measuring a patient's affective or cognitive response to an intervention, one clearly is dealing with process, but also with immediate outcome if the response is rated along a positive-negative dimension. A positive immediate outcome might involve increased productivity and accessing of memories, dreams, or fantasies, whereas a negative immediate outcome might be indicated by patient defensiveness.

Outcome Research

Paradoxically, the impetus for psychotherapy research began with Eysenck's (1952) finding that a control group and a treated group of neurotic patients did equally well. Eysenck claimed that two-thirds of patients improved substantially within 2 years, regardless of whether they received treatment. A number of methodological problems were found in Eysenck's work, casting doubt on his findings. However, Eysenck's criticism spawned a host of psychotherapy research, culminating in the Smith et al. (1980) meta-analysis. Meta-analysis involves a systematic search of the literature to identify studies meeting specific inclusion criteria. It provides a quantitative summary of a large number of studies by employing a common measure, such as effect size. In their analysis of 475 clinical trials, Smith and colleagues found that the average person receiving treatment was better off than 80% of untreated control subjects (average effect size = 0.85).

A number of meta-analytic reviews of outcome in anxiety disorders and depression have been conducted. Clum (1989) identified 283 studies involving panic or agoraphobia patients treated with behavior therapy. Seventy percent of the treated patients improved, compared with 30% of the untreated control subjects. Dobson (1989), examining 10 studies of patients with depression treated with cognitive therapy, reported that the average treated patient was better off than 98% of the untreated patients (i.e., an effect size of 2.15). Robinson et al. (1990) identified 29 studies in which depressed patients were treated with either cognitive-behavioral or general verbal therapies (client-centered, dynamic, and interpersonal). All treatments produced a positive outcome compared with no treatment or a waiting-list control condition (effect size = 0.84), and there were no differences in efficacy among the different treatments.

In a review of the effectiveness of psychotherapy for personality disorders, J. C. Perry et al. (1999) identified 15 studies that reported treatment outcomes in this patient population. The treatments used included psychodynamic-interpersonal, cognitive-behavioral, mixed, and supportive therapies. They concluded that psychotherapy is an effective treatment for personality disorders (effect sizes were 1.11 for self-report measures and

1.29 for observational measures). It should be noted that some of the treatments were relatively long-term (up to 25.4 months). Patients with borderline or other more severe types of personality disorders tended to receive longer-duration treatments, usually dynamic in nature.

In the National Institute of Mental Health (NIMH) Treatment of Depression Collaborative Research Program (Elkin et al. 1989; Elkin 1994; Imber et al. 1990), two different psychotherapies—cognitive-behavioral therapy (CBT) and interpersonal therapy (IPT)—were compared with an antidepressant (imipramine)–clinical management condition and a control condition consisting of drug placebo and clinical management. The clinical management was a low-level supportive approach. This study was important in that it attempted to deliver a standardized and competently conducted treatment for depression by using therapy manuals with adherence ratings. Although both psychotherapies were effective, there were essentially no significant differences between CBT and IPT on measures of depressive symptoms, overall functioning, or mode-specific effects. In addition, there was a general lack of significant differences between either of the psychotherapies and the placebo–clinical management condition.

In another study of depression, Shapiro et al. (1994) treated 117 patients (stratified by illness severity) with 8 or 16 sessions of either cognitive-behavioral or psychodynamic-interpersonal psychotherapy. They found the two treatments to be equally effective on most measures, except that one depression inventory indicated some advantage for cognitive-behavioral treatment. An interesting finding was that patients with relatively severe depression demonstrated more improvement after 16 sessions than after 8 sessions. This result suggests that severity of illness may be an important factor in determining the optimal length of treatment, even within a short-term framework. A follow-up assessment of this group of patients 1 year after they completed treatment revealed some changes in the findings (Shapiro et al. 1995). Patients who received 8-session psychodynamic-interpersonal therapy had maintained their improvement less well than those who received either 16-session psychodynamic-interpersonal therapy or cognitive-behavioral therapy of 8 or 16 sessions. In addition, 16-session cognitive-behavioral treatment no longer showed an advantage over 8-session treatment, even when severity of illness was taken into account.

In a meta-analysis of 11 studies in which short-term dynamic psychotherapy was employed, Crits-Christoph (1992) reported effect sizes significantly greater for short-term dynamic psychotherapy than for the waiting-list control condition. The 11 studies included patients with depression, personality disorders, posttraumatic stress disorder, pathological grief, opiate addiction, and cocaine abuse. Some of the studies compared short-term dynamic psychotherapy with other psychotherapies and with nonpsychiatric treatments such as support groups. No significant differences were found between various psychotherapies and other psychiatric treatments or even nonpsychiatric treatments.

A. Winston and colleagues (1994a) compared two forms of brief dynamic therapy with a waiting-list control condition in patients with Cluster C personality disorders (i.e., obsessive-compulsive, avoidant, dependent). One therapy was cognitively based, and the other used a confrontational, affect-focused approach. They found significant improvement in both treatment conditions as compared with the waiting-list condition. Again, the two therapies did not differ in overall outcome.

In two other studies in personality disorder patients that contrasted interpretative and supportive forms of psychotherapy, both therapies produced improvement, and patient outcomes were equivalent (Hellerstein et al. 1998; Piper et al. 1998). In the first study, by Hellerstein et al. (1998), patients had personality disorders primarily of the Cluster C type, and nearly all had Axis I comorbidity as well. In the second study, that of Piper et al. (1998), all patients had an Axis I diagnosis, generally a mood or anxiety disorder, and approximately 60% also had an Axis II disorder.

A number of meta-analyses and reviews (Lambert and Bergin 1994; Luborsky et al. 1975; Smith et al. 1980; Rachman and Wilson 1980) also have concluded that there are no significant differences between psychotherapies. These studies indicate that psychotherapy is effective, but that evidence for the superiority of a particular model of psychotherapy is not readily apparent for many disorders. Luborsky and colleagues (1975) elaborated on Rosenzweig's (1936) use of the "Dodo bird verdict," calling attention to the lack of significant outcome differences between therapies. (In *Alice in Wonderland,* the Dodo bird exclaims, "Everyone has won and all must have prizes.") The Dodo bird verdict was challenged by Beutler (1991), who argued that it is premature to abandon the search for differential effects. He cited two major problems contributing to the failure to identify Patient × Psychotherapy interaction effects (Beutler 1991, p. 226): 1) "an unmanageably large number of patient and treatment variables that potentially interact with one another," and 2) the fact that "many theoretically important constructs in psychotherapy lack either consensual or consistent meaning." Beutler concluded by stressing the necessity for a "guiding framework that leads to both differential hypotheses and differential clinical decisions."

We believe that the study of an integrated model of psychotherapy, matching different procedures with a variety of patient characteristics, can offer the potential of finding differential effects.

Evidence based on systematic research is beginning to emerge that suggests the superiority of specific psychotherapies for certain Axis I disorders. For example, cognitive-behavioral treatment appears to be the most efficacious psychotherapy for panic disorder (Barlow and Craske 1989; Clark and Salkovskis 1989) and simple phobias (Smith et al. 1980). Specific interventions employed in CBT include cognitive restructuring, (interoceptive) exposure, progressive muscle relaxation, and breathing retraining. Behavior therapy, using exposure therapy and response prevention, has clear advantages over other approaches for obsessive-compulsive disorder (Foa et al. 1984, 1985; Greist 1990; Marks 1986). Posttraumatic stress disorder appears to respond well to exposure therapy, stress inoculation training, or the combination of both (Foa 1997; Foa et al. 1991). Finally, a combined approach using exposure and cognitive restructuring appears to be highly effective for social phobia (Hope and Heimberg 1993; Mattick and Peters 1988; Mattick et al. 1989).

Reasons for Lack of Significant Differences in Outcome Among Therapies

The lack of significant differences in outcome among therapies has been attributed to a number of factors. These include therapist variables, heterogeneous patient populations, high improvement rates, measurement issues, premature patient termination, and common factors across psychotherapies or schools of psychotherapy.

Therapist Factors

To begin with, it is well known that therapists vary in therapeutic ability (Lafferty et al. 1989; Lambert 1989; Luborsky et al. 1986; Luborsky et al. 1993; Orlinsky and Howard 1980). If studies do not control for these differences, methodological problems can result. Attempts have been made to match therapists and patients on global personality dimensions such as psychological differentiation (Pardes et al. 1974), personality type (Whitehorn and Betz 1960), and others (Antonuccio et al. 1982; Mendelson and Geller 1967). These attempts have not proven to be worthwhile (Talley et al. 1990; Tuma et al. 1978). Dougherty (1976) and Parloff et al. (1978) concluded that little evidence exists that either similarity or dissimilarity of patient and therapist personality styles is consistently associated with patient improvement. However, assessment of the interpersonal styles of psychotherapists during psychotherapy may be a more productive approach. Circumplex models of interpersonal interactions have been used to study patient-therapist compatibility (Wiggins 1982), an approach discussed later in this chapter.

Heterogeneity of Patient Populations

A second possible reason for the lack of differences in outcome observed between therapies is the heterogeneity of the patient population studied. Patients vary in many ways across a large number of variables, including demographics, diagnosis, and defensive and interpersonal styles (Beutler 1991). Many brief psychotherapies are employed in the treatment of patients with personality disorders (such as dependent, avoidant, obsessive-compulsive, passive-aggressive, histrionic, and mixed types). These diagnostic categories are extremely difficult to diagnose reliably, which may further confound outcome results with these patients. The use of dimensional rather than categorical approaches may yield more productive outcome data (Frances et al. 1990). This means that research would address personality dimensions such as dependence, avoidance, and masochistic behavior across diagnostic categories instead of simply using current personality disorder diagnosis.

High Improvement Rates

A third possible reason for the inability of studies to detect significant differences in outcome among therapies is the high improvement rates observed in much of the research. Given that most studies of brief psychotherapy report that the vast majority (approximately 70%) of patients improve significantly, little room exists for differences to be demonstrated (Crits-Christoph 1992; Elkin et al. 1989; Foa et al. 1991; Smith et al. 1980; A. Winston et al. 1994a). This problem is magnified in studies with small numbers of patients, a characteristic that unfortunately applies to the majority of psychotherapy studies. Collaborative studies among multiple centers can provide larger numbers of subjects so that smaller differences might become apparent (Luborsky et al. 1993). Severity of illness is another factor that may be related to small sample size (McLellan et al. 1983). Most psychotherapies are effective in healthier patients and much less effective in severely ill patients. This leaves a middle group of patients in whom differences might be found.

An innovative approach to the problem/dilemma of high improvement rates is found in the work of Piper and colleagues (1998). These researchers stratified patients on the dimension of quality of object relations (QOR), comparing supportive and interpretive psychotherapies. They found a direct relationship between QOR and outcome with interpretive therapy but almost no relationship between QOR and outcome with supportive therapy. This result suggests that the patients with low QOR may have been less able to tolerate the demands of interpretive therapy as opposed to supportive psychotherapy, where the level of tension is kept low and fewer demands are made on the patient.

Measurement Issues

Measurement issues may be another factor contributing to the similarity of results across therapies. Many investigators have suggested the need for more sensitive and comprehensive outcome measures (Luborsky et al. 1993). For example, indicators of dynamic change, such as insight, are particularly difficult to measure. A number of studies have relied only on symptomatic change, a measure that may not completely capture the nuances of how therapies differ in their effects on cognition, long-term problem solving, and self-object representations.

Premature Patient Termination

Yet another important measurement issue is that of patient withdrawal from psychotherapy studies. Premature patient termination occurs fairly often. Wierzbicki and Pekarik (1993) reported a 46.86% mean dropout rate in their meta-analysis of 125 studies. An "intention to treat" approach is a somewhat newer methodology in which dropouts are included in the outcome analysis by obtaining outcome data from all subjects, not just those completing treatment. Use of intention-to-treat models may aid in the effort to find outcome differences among therapies.

A more intensive examination of premature patient termination as well as treatment failure may shed light on the various factors contributing to a lack of success in psychotherapy. In a recent study of patients who dropped out of short-term psychotherapy treatment or had poor outcomes, Samstag and colleagues (1998) were able to identify a number of predictive variables during the early phase of treatment. These variables included patient- and therapist-rated measures of the quality of the therapeutic alliance and interpersonal process. Patients who dropped out had evidence of a poor therapeutic alliance and in-session expression of hostility. Therapist attention to such issues early in treatment may lead to improved outcomes.

Common Factors

The most important reason for lack of differences in overall outcome between psychotherapies may relate to the fact that all psychotherapeutic approaches share certain common elements. These common elements may play a major role in patient improvement and may have a large effect size in comparison with the more technical or specific factors that characterize different treatments. Although these technical differences undoubtedly affect outcome, it may be that their influence is small compared with the common factors. Rosenzweig (1936), Frank and Frank (1991), and Lambert (1986) have described key elements of the common factors, which can be organized into six components (A. Winston and Muran 1996):

1. Expression of feelings and thoughts (Rosenzweig 1936)
2. Self-examination and self-understanding (Rosenzweig 1936)
3. Provision of a rationale that includes a plausible system of explanation of the patient's problems or distress (Frank and Frank 1991)
4. Strengthening the patient's expectations of help—the arousal of hope (Frank and Frank 1991)
5. Encouragement of mastery efforts and testing of different approaches and solutions (Lambert 1986)
6. The patient-therapist or helping relationship (Frank and Frank 1991)

These six common factors were discussed in Chapter 5. Of these, the sixth factor, the patient-therapist relationship, may be the most important (Hartley 1985; Horvath and Symonds 1991; A. Winston and Muran 1996). Strupp (1995) stated that the nature of the therapeutic relationship is the sine qua non in all psychotherapies. Because of the central position and overriding importance of this factor, we will examine research involving the patient-therapist relationship in greater detail in the following section.

Process Research

Process research linked to outcome is designed to identify process variables that may be therapeutic, nontherapeutic, or even harmful. The overall aim is to determine which interventions are useful in producing change under what circumstances and clinical situations. In this section we focus on the therapeutic relationship and the interpersonal process between patient and therapist, which we believe is the paramount issue in process research.

The Patient-Therapist Relationship

Freud's (1912/1958) early theoretical papers on transference called attention to the importance of the patient-therapist relationship. Greenson (1967) suggested that the therapeutic relationship consists of three components: a transference-countertransference configuration, a real relationship, and a working alliance. Although these components were discussed separately in Chapter 4 to promote clarity, we believe that they are intimately connected. Accordingly, in this chapter we use the terms *therapeutic relationship* and *patient-therapist relationship* synonymously to refer to a single entity that encompasses all three components, unless we are focusing on a specific aspect of the relationship, such as the therapeutic alliance.

Clinicians have long recognized the centrality of the therapeutic relationship and the importance of working within this relationship. The innovators of brief dynamic psychotherapy (Davanloo 1980; Malan 1976, 1979; Sifneos 1972) paid a great deal of attention to the patient-therapist relationship and the need to link a patient's behavior toward the therapist to significant individuals in the patient's life. Indeed, exploration of the here-and-now of the relationship can have great therapeutic value because of the immediacy of these issues as they unfold between the participants (Gill 1979). The interpersonal and object relations theorists (J. Greenberg and Mitchell 1983) stressed the importance of the therapeutic relationship and described psychological development in a relational context. The significance of the therapeutic relationship also was noted by cognitive (Safran and Segal 1990) and behavioral writers (R.J. Kohlenberg and Tsai 1991).

The Therapeutic Alliance

The patient-therapist relationship has been most thoroughly studied using the concept of the therapeutic alliance. Most investigators consider the alliance to reflect the ability of patient and therapist to work purposefully together in treatment and the quality of the affective bond between them. A number of assessment scales have been developed to examine various aspects of the alliance from the patient's, therapist's, and/or observer's perspective. Luborsky (1976) developed the Penn Helping Alliance Scale (HAQ), which was later tested in patients treated with brief dynamic therapy using two raters (Luborsky et al. 1983). The first empirical study of the alliance in psychotherapy employed the Vanderbilt Psychotherapy Process Scale (VPPS), as rated by two judges (Gomes-Schwartz 1978). Other measures developed to study the alliance include the Vanderbilt Therapeutic Alliance Scale (VTAS; Hartley and Strupp 1983), the California Psychotherapy Alliance Scales (CALPAS; Marmar et al. 1989), and the Working Alliance Inventory (WAI; Horvath and Greenberg 1989, 1994). Selected items from the California Psychotherapy Alliance Scale—Patient Version are presented in Table 10–1.

In a review of research on the therapeutic alliance in psychotherapy, Hartley (1985) found that patient ratings of the alliance were more highly correlated with outcome than were therapist ratings and that ratings made early in treatment were highly correlated with outcome. Gaston (1990), writing on different aspects of the alliance, concluded that the concept of the alliance was theoretically sound and clinically useful and that empirical

---

TABLE 10–1. Selected items from the four factors of the California Psychotherapy Alliance Scale—Patient Version

Patient commitment

Did you feel that even if you might have moments of doubts, confusion, or mistrust, overall therapy is worthwhile?

How much did you find yourself thinking that therapy was not the best way to get help with your problems?

Patient working capacity

When important things come to mind, how often did you find yourself keeping them to yourself rather than sharing them with your therapist?

How much did you hold back your feelings during this session?

Therapist understanding and involvement

Did you feel accepted and respected by your therapist for who you are?

During this session, how dedicated was your therapist to helping you overcome your difficulties?

Working strategy consensus

Did you feel that you were working together with your therapist, that the two of you were joined in a struggle to overcome your problems?

Did the treatment you received in this session match with your ideas about what helps people in therapy?

Source. Adapted from Gaston 1991.

---

evidence supported its predictive validity in psychotherapy outcome. Finally, in a meta-analysis of 24 studies of different psychotherapies, Horvath and Symonds (1991) found a moderate but reliable association between a good working alliance and positive outcome. The therapies examined included cognitive, dynamic, gestalt, and eclectic or mixed therapies. No significant differences were observed between the type of therapy and the relationship between alliance and outcome. Horvath and Symonds also found that patient ratings were more predictive than either therapist or observer assessments.

Hatcher and Barends (1996) used three alliance measures (HAQ, CALPAS, and WAI) to study patients' perceptions of the alliance in psychodynamic psychotherapy. They found that the dimension most emphasized by patients was the "Confident Collaboration factor, which expresses the [patient's] sense of committed participation in a helpful, hopeful process with the therapist" (Hatcher and Barends 1996, p. 1334). Greenson (1967) stressed the collaborative nature of the alliance and the "patient's capacity to work purposively in the treatment situation" (p. 192). Bordin (1979) also highlighted the joint effort of patient and therapist and the patient's active involvement in the work of therapy. Thus, working effectively with the therapist plays a central role in the action of the therapeutic alliance.

Stiles et al. (1998), using the Agnew Relationship Measure (ARM), studied the therapeutic alliance in patients with depression treated with time-limited psychodynamic-interpersonal or cognitive-behavioral therapies. They found that gains on outcome measures were associated with higher ARM scores, with alliance measured later in therapy, and with alliances that increased as therapy progressed. Interestingly, the ARM subscale that best correlated with outcome was similar to Hatcher and Barends' Confidence Collaborative factor.

Attempts to characterize the mechanism by which the alliance effects change have yielded two models: 1) the alliance as a precondition or matrix for change and 2) the alliance as the actual agent of change. Light has been shed on this issue by a number of investigators who have examined the alliance at various points over the course of therapy. Some studies have found that the alliance is stable across therapy and that the quality of the alliance as assessed early in treatment is the best predictor of outcome (Horvath and Symonds 1991; Muran et al. 1997). This finding is consistent with the alliance as a precondition or foundation for improvement (i.e., the first mechanism cited above). Other studies have demonstrated that improvement in the alliance over the course of treatment is associated with good outcome (Foreman and Marmar 1985; Luborsky et al. 1993). These results tend to favor the notion that the alliance is the actual change agent for improvement in therapy (i.e., the second mechanism cited above).

In a study of two forms of brief dynamic therapy, Westerman et al. (1995) suggested that the question of which of the two proposed mechanisms applies may depend on which treatment is studied. For short-term dynamic psychotherapy (Davanloo 1980; Laikin et al. 1991), they found that improvement in the alliance over the course of treatment was associated with good outcome, a result favoring the notion of the alliance as change agent. For brief adaptive psychotherapy (Pollack et al. 1991), however, outcome was related to the quality of the early alliance, and change in alliance from the beginning to the end of therapy was not related to improvement, a finding consistent with the alliance as the foundation for successful treatment. The proposed explanation for this finding is that short-term dynamic psychotherapy emphasizes consistent and systematic exploration of the here-and-now of the patient-therapist relationship, whereas brief adaptive psychotherapy does not focus as much or as consistently on the relationship. One clinical implication of this study is that a flexible approach should be productive in maintaining or improving the therapeutic alliance. In cases in which the alliance is initially poor, immediate, rapid, and intensive therapeutic exploration of the patient-therapist relationship might be required. On the other hand, in situations in which an early positive therapeutic alliance has been established, the therapeutic relationship might not need to be systematically addressed.

Ruptures in the Alliance

Research evidence is clear and consistent in finding the alliance to be an important variable in mediating treatment outcome. However, very little research has examined the factors involved in establishing and maintaining a good alliance or repairing a problematic one. Research on resolving ruptures in the therapeutic alliance is a major focus of the Beth Israel Brief Psychotherapy Program in New York City (Safran and Muran 1998, 2000; Safran et al. 1994). Two types of ruptures have been delineated: confrontation and withdrawal. These represent contrasting ways of coping with the tension between the need for relatedness and the need for self-definition. In confrontation ruptures, the need for self-definition is stronger than that for relatedness. In withdrawal ruptures, relatedness takes precedence over self-definition (Safran and Muran 2000). The process of identifying and resolving ruptures offers valuable opportunities to learn about internal mental processes and facilitate patient change. (For a more complete discussion of rupture resolution, see Chapter 4.)

Factors Contributing to the Alliance

Patient Personality

Patient and therapist personality factors and their interaction in psychotherapy should play a major role in how the therapeutic alliance develops. Unfortunately, research findings in this area are somewhat limited, conflicting, and uninformative. Some investigators (Marmar et al. 1986; Marziali 1984; Piper et al. 1991) have found patient interpersonal functioning to be significantly related to the quality of the alliance, while others (Gaston et al. 1988) have found no such relationship. Moras and Strupp's (1982) findings were mixed: they reported that although good pretreatment interpersonal functioning of patients predicted a good alliance, poor interpersonal functioning did not predict a poor alliance. Unfortunately, these studies used a single, unidimensional index of interpersonal functioning by considering all interpersonal problems in a global fashion. Research evidence indicates that interpersonal behavior is multidimensional in nature (Wiggins 1982) and that some interpersonal behaviors may have more detrimental effects on the alliance than others.

Another approach to the study of interpersonal problems involves the use of the two-dimensional circumplex models of interpersonal behavior (Wiggins 1982) (see Figure 10–1). Circumplex models arrange interpersonal behavior on a surface defined by two axes. The horizontal axis represents the affective or affiliative dimension and has end points such as friendliness and hostility or warm and cold. The vertical axis represents the power or control dimension and has end points such as dominance and submission. Muran et al. (1994), using an interpersonal circumplex interpretation, found that hostile-dominant problems were negatively related and overly friendly–submissive problems positively related to the development of aspects of the alliance for patients in short-term cognitive therapy. A. Winston et al. (1994b) reported similar results for patients in dynamic psychotherapy. These results are consistent with the findings of Horowitz and colleagues, who reported that patients with friendly-submissive interpersonal styles had better outcomes in short-term psychotherapy (L. M. Horowitz et al. 1993).

Circumplex models also have been used to assess the degree of fit of the behaviors of two people in a dyadic interaction. A great deal of evidence has accrued to indicate that a correspondence on affiliation by therapist and patient (e.g., patient-friendly and therapist-friendly; Orford 1986) is predictive of both the quality of the therapeutic alliance and the treatment outcome (Henry et al. 1986; Muran et al. 1997)

Therapist Personality

Little has been reported in the research literature about the effect of the therapist's personality on the alliance. The Vanderbilt Psychotherapy Studies, using manualized therapy, showed that therapists had limited success with patients who entered therapy with attitudes of negativism, hostility, and resistance (Strupp 1993). When the cases of patients with poor outcomes were examined, it was found that some of the therapists engaged in high levels of conflicted interpersonal processes, such as interpretations made in a subtly blaming manner or "supportive" statements that conveyed a criticism of the patient. In a study examining the effects of an extensive training program designed to change therapists' behavior, Henry et al. (1993) reported some improvement in therapists' technical interventions after the training, but found that therapists with self-reported hostile and controlling introjects still engaged in greater frequencies of countertherapeutic interpersonal processes,

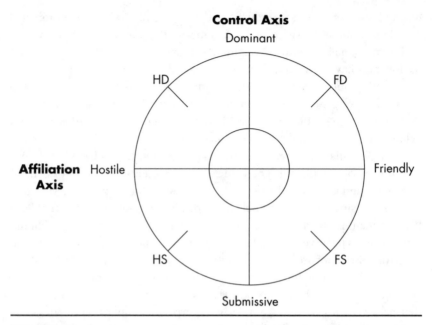

FIGURE 10–1. Interpersonal circumplex model. HD = hostile-dominant; FD = friendly-dominant; HS = hostile-submissive; FS = friendly-submissive.
Source. Wiggins 1982.

such as negative or complex communications. Even after training, these therapists were judged to be less approving and supportive, less optimistic, and more authoritative and defensive than other therapists. Henry and colleagues concluded that "traditional training may more easily change surface features of therapists' behavior, with less impact on the interpersonal 'deep structure' of the therapeutic relationship" (p. 439).

The findings of Strupp (1993) and Henry et al. (1993) call into question the use of therapy manuals, particularly those manuals that are highly prescriptive. Therapists need to be able to be flexible with patients and not rigidly adhere to an approach that may not be suited for a patient. An integrated psychotherapy using techniques best suited to the patient, within a framework that emphasizes maintaining and strengthening the therapeutic relationship, may be the best approach with difficult patients.

Patient-Therapist Interactions

Examinations of specific patient or therapist variables have not revealed any significant relationships with outcome. However, certain key patient-therapist interactional sequences appear to offer a better chance to understand patient change. The study of recurring episodes of patient and therapist interactions was undertaken by McCullough and colleagues (1991). These studies involved patients with personality disorders (primarily of the Cluster C group) treated with two types of brief dynamic psychotherapy. All sessions were videotaped, and four of the sessions, one from each quartile of treatment, were then coded for therapist clarifications, transference interpretations, and nontransference interpretations followed by patient defensive behavior or affect. Outcome at 1 month after termination demonstrated significant clinical improvement with both therapies, with an effect size of 1.0 (A. Winston et al. 1991). Results of the process study revealed that transference interpretations followed by patient affect were strongly correlated with positive outcome, whereas a composite of therapist interventions followed by patient defensive behavior were correlated with poor outcome. Thus, an emergence of affect—as opposed to a rise in defensive behavior—in response to therapist interventions appears to be an important clinical marker for eventual success in brief dynamic psychotherapy.

Conclusions

We have presented a brief review of outcome and process psychotherapy research. Efficacy studies of brief psychotherapy indicate that approximately 70% of patients improve significantly. More research is needed to understand which psychotherapy or combination of psychotherapies will best address a specific disorder, problem, or situation. Eventually we should be able to determine which approach is best for an individual patient by using a system of differential therapeutics.

For the 30% of patients for whom treatment is not effective, more intensive process research will be helpful in identifying effective change agents. One promising area of study is the work on the therapeutic alliance and alliance rupture resolution (Safran and Muran 2000).

In Conclusion

Use of a single psychotherapeutic approach no longer appears appropriate. Patients present with a wide variety of symptoms, personality patterns, conflicts, affects, defenses, and coping abilities. Comorbidity is quite common, so that it is not unusual for individuals to have both mood and anxiety disorders as well as personality disorders. Cognitive-behavioral therapy is the treatment of choice for many mood and anxiety disorders, whereas dynamic/interpersonal psychotherapy is indicated for conflicts and interpersonal problems. Because many patients have various combinations of disorders and problems, an approach that integrates a number of treatments and a range of interventions has a clear advantage over a unidimensional approach.

We have presented a framework for the integration of multiple approaches. Beginning with the concept of a continuum of psychopathology (health-sickness) that is superimposed on another continuum of dynamic psychotherapy, a range of interventions can be used that fit the needs and level of psychopathology of the patient. The therapeutic approach can be as supportive as necessary for patients with severe psychopathology, or more exploratory (expressive) for healthier individuals. Cognitive-behavioral techniques are used for such problems as depressive and anxiety disorders as well as for dysfunctional thinking. Interpersonal and relational models are incorporated into the integrated approach to address problems in these areas.

The use of the therapeutic relationship will vary depending on the patient's placement on the continuum. For patients in supportive/cognitive-behavioral therapy, patient-therapist relationship issues are noted and monitored but are generally not explored unless they are clearly problematic. Individuals in expressive treatment will generally benefit from an exploration of the therapeutic relationship.

A treatment that is truly integrated will use medication when indicated. Not all patients require medication, but many do better with a combined approach of psychotherapy and medication. Using a combined approach requires therapists to be knowledgeable about the indications for introducing medication into psychotherapy.

Therapists should have a working knowledge of the approaches discussed in this book and should be able to transition from one approach to another. Such transitioning involves combining various interventions from different psychotherapy traditions into a cohesive therapy. To accomplish this requires a great deal of therapist flexibility and firsthand knowledge of a number of therapies. It is important to begin to train therapists who can provide an integrated treatment.

The integrated model presented here can be applied to both time-limited and time-unlimited therapy. In this book we have focused on brief psychotherapy, which is efficacious for a wide variety of patients. A major challenge for our field is to continue developing brief therapies that will help patients within a reasonable time frame and at the same time integrate a number of therapeutic approaches and interventions to provide optimum treatment.

References

Alexander F: Current views on psychotherapy. Psychiatry 16:113–122, 1953

Alexander F: The dynamics of psychotherapy in the light of learning theory. Am J Psychiatry 120:440–448, 1963

Alexander F, French TM: Psychoanalytic Psychotherapy. New York, Ronald Press, 1946

Angst J: Major depression in 1998: are we providing optimal care? J Clin Psychiatry 60 (suppl 6):5–9, 1999

Angst J, Baastrup P, Grof P, et al: The course of monopolar depression and bipolar psychoses. Psychiatr Neurol Neurochir 76:489–500, 1973

Antonuccio DO, Lewinsohn PM, Steinmetz JL: Identification of therapist differences in group treatment for depression. J Consult Clin Psychol 50:433–435, 1982

Arlow J: Fantasy, memory, and reality testing. Psychoanalytic Quarterly 38:28–51, 1969

Aron L: A Meeting of Minds. Hillsdale, NJ, Analytic Press, 1996

Baker HS, Baker MN: Heinz Kohut's self psychology: an overview. Am J Psychiatry 144:1–9, 1987

Balint M, Ornstein PH, Balint E: Focal Psychotherapy: An Example of Applied Psychoanalysis. London, Tavistock, 1972

Bandura A: Self-efficiency mechanisms in human agency. Am Psychol 37:122–147, 1982

Barlow D: Anxiety and Its Disorders: The Nature and Treatment of Anxiety and Panic. New York, Guilford, 1988

Barlow D, Craske M: Mastery of Your Anxiety and Panic. Albany, NY, Center for Stress and Anxiety Disorders, State University of New York, 1989

Battle C, Imber S, Hoehn-Saric R, et al: Target complaints as a criteria of improvement. Am J Psychotherapy 20:184–192, 1966

Beck AT: Thinking and depression, I: idiosyncratic content and cognitive distortions. Arch Gen Psychiatry 9:324–333, 1963

Beck AT: Depression: Clinical, Experimental and Theoretical Aspects. New York, Hoeber, 1967

Beck AT: Cognitive Therapy and the Emotional Disorders. New York, International Universities Press, 1976

Beck AT, Rush AJ, Shaw BF, et al: Cognitive Therapy of Depression: A Treatment Manual. New York, Guilford, 1979

Beitman BD: Pharmacotherapy as an intervention during the stages of psychotherapy. Am J Psychother 35:206–214, 1981

Beitman BD, Chiles J, Carlin A: The pharmacotherapy-psychotherapy triangle: psychiatrist, non-medical psychotherapist, and patient. J Clin Psychiatry 45:458–459, 1984

Bellak L: The schizophrenic syndrome: a further elaboration of the unified theory of schizophrenia, in Schizophrenia: A Review of the Syndrome. New York, Logos, 1958, pp 3–63

Benton MK, Schroeder HE: Social skills training with schizophrenics: a meta-analytic evaluation. J Consult Clin Psychol 58:741–747, 1990

Beres D: Ego deviation and the concept of schizophrenia. The Psychoanalytic Study of the Child, Vol 11. New York, International Universities Press, 1956, pp 164–235

Beutler LE: Have all won and must all have prizes? Revisiting Luborsky et al.'s verdict. J Consult Clin Psychol 39:226–232, 1991

Binstock WA: Prescribing psychotherapy, in Outpatient Psychiatry: Diagnosis and Treatment. Edited by Lazare A. Baltimore, MD, Williams & Wilkins, 1979, pp 603-611

Blackburn IM, Bishop S, Glen AIM, et al: The efficacy of cognitive therapy in depression: a treatment trial using cognitive and pharmacotherapy, each alone and in combination. Br J Psychiatry 139:181–189, 1981

Blagys MD, Hilsenroth MJ: Distinctive features of short-term psychodynamic-interpersonal psychotherapy: a review of the comparative psychotherapy process literature. Clinical Psychology: Science and Practice 7:167–188, 2000

Blanck G, Blanck R: Ego Psychology: Theory and Practice. New York, Columbia University Press, 1974

Bond GR, McGrew JH, Fekete DM: Assertive outreach for frequent users of psychiatric hospitals: a meta-analysis. J Ment Health Adm 22:4–16, 1995

Bordin ES: The generalizability of the psychoanalytic concept of the working alliance. Psychotherapy: Theory, Research, and Practice 16:252–260, 1979

Breuer J, Freud S: Studies on hysteria (1893–1895), in The Standard Edition of the Complete Psychological Works of Sigmund Freud, Vol 2. Edited by Strachey J. London, Hogarth Press, 1955, pp 3–181

Bromberg P: On knowing one's patient inside out. Psychoanalytic Dialogues 1:399–422, 1991

Brown GR, Anderson B: Psychiatric morbidity in adult inpatients with childhood histories of sexual and physical abuse. Am J Psychiatry 148:55–61, 1993

Butler SF, Strupp HH: Specific and nonspecific factors in psychotherapy: a problematic paradigm for psychotherapy research. Psychotherapy 23:30–40, 1986

Carli T: The psychologically informed psychopharmacologist, in Psychopharmacology and Psychotherapy: A Collaborative Approach. Edited by Riba MB, Balon R. Washington, DC, American Psychiatric Press, 1999, pp 179–196

Carroll KM: Integrating psychotherapy and pharmacotherapy to improve drug abuse outcomes. Addict Behav 22:233–245, 1997

Carroll KM, Nich C, Rounsaville BJ: Differential symptom reduction in depressed cocaine abusers treated with psychotherapy and pharmacotherapy. J Nerv Ment Dis 183:251–259, 1995

Charney DS, Nelson CJ: Delusional and nondelusional unipolar depression: further evidence for distinct types. Am J Psychiatry 138:328–333, 1981

Clark DM, Salkovskis P: Cognitive Treatment of Panic and Hypochondrias. New York, Pergamon, 1989

Clarkin JF, Glick ID, Haas GL, et al: A randomized clinical trial of inpatient family intervention, V: results for affective disorders. J Affect Disord 18:17–28, 1990

Clum GA: Psychological interventions vs drugs in the treatment of panic. Behavior Therapy 20:429–457, 1989

Cochran SD: Preventing medical noncompliance in the outpatient treatment of bipolar affective disorders. J Consult Clin Psychol 52:873–878, 1984

Conte HR, Plutchik R, Wild KV, et al: Combined psychotherapy and pharmacotherapy for depression. A systematic analysis of the evidence. Arch Gen Psychiatry 43:471–479, 1986

Crits-Christoph P: The efficacy of brief dynamic psychotherapy: a meta-analysis. Am J Psychiatry 149:151–158, 1992

Davanloo H: A method of short-term dynamic psychotherapy, in Short-Term Dynamic Psychotherapy. Edited by Davanloo H. Northvale NJ, Jason Aronson, 1980, pp 43–71

Depression Guideline Panel, Agency for Health Care Policy and Research: Depression in Primary Care, Vol 2: Treatment of Major Depression. Clinical Practice Guidelines, Number 5 (AHCPR publication 93-0551). Rockville, MD, Department of Health and Human Services, U.S. Public Health Service, 1993

DeRubeis RJ, Beck AT: Cognitive therapy, in Handbook of Cognitive-Behavioral Therapies. Edited by Dobson KS. New York, Guilford, 1988, pp 273–306

Dewald PA: Psychotherapy: A Dynamic Approach. New York, Basic Books, 1971

Dewan M: Are psychiatrists cost-effective? An analysis of integrated versus split treatment. Am J Psychiatry 156:324–326, 1999

Dobson KS: A meta-analysis of the efficacy of cognitive therapy for depression. J Consult Clin Psychol 57:414–419, 1989

Dobson KS, Block L: Historical and philosophical basis of the cognitive-behavioral therapies, in Handbook of Cognitive-Behavioral Therapies. Edited by Dobson KS. New York, Guilford, 1988, pp 3–38

Dougherty FE: Patient-therapist matching for prediction of optimal and minimal therapeutic outcome. J Consult Clin Psychol 44:889–897, 1976

Elkin I: The NIMH Treatment of Depression Collaborative Research Program: where we began and where we are, in Handbook of Psychotherapy and Behavior Change. Edited by Bergin AE, Garfield SL. New York, Wiley, 1994, pp 114–139

Elkin I, Shea MT, Watkins JT, et al: National Institute of Mental Health Treatment of Depression Collaborative Research Program. General effectiveness of treatments. Arch Gen Psychiatry 46:971–983, 1989

Ellis A: Reason and Emotion in Psychotherapy. Secaucus, NJ, Lyle Stuart, 1962

Ellis A: The history of cognition in psychotherapy, in Comprehensive Handbook of Cognitive Therapy. Edited by Freeman A, Simon KM, Beutler LE, et al. New York, Plenum, 1989, pp 5–19

Emde RN: Positive emotions for psychoanalytic theory: surprises from infancy research and new directions, in Affect: Psychoanalytic Perspectives. Edited by Shapiro T, Emde RN. Madison, CT, International Universities Press, 1992, pp 5–44

Erikson EH: Childhood and Society. New York, WW Norton, 1950

Eysenck HJ: The effects of psychotherapy: an evaluation. Journal of Consulting Psychology 16:319–324, 1952

Fairbairn WRD: An Object-Relations Theory of the Personality. New York, Basic Books, 1952

Ferenczi S: The further development of an active therapy in psychoanalysis (1921), in Further Contributions to the Theory and Technique of Psychoanalysis. Edited by Suttie J. London, Karnac Books, 1980, pp 189–197

Ferenczi S, Rank O: The Development of Psychoanalysis (1925). Translated by Newton C. New York, Dover, 1956

Foa EB: Trauma and women: course, predictors, and treatment. J Clin Psychiatry 58:25–28, 1997

Foa EB, Steketee G, Grayson JB, et al: Deliberate exposure and blocking of obsessive-compulsive rituals: immediate and long-term effects. Behavior Therapy 15:450–472, 1984

Foa EB, Steketee G, Ozarow B: Behavior therapy with obsessive-compulsives: from theory to treatment, in Obsessive-Compulsive Disorder: Psychological and Pharmacological Treatment. Edited by Mavissakalian M. New York, Plenum, 1985

Foa EB, Rothbaum BO, Riggs DS, et al: Treatment of posttraumatic stress disorder in rape victims: a comparison between cognitive-behavioral procedures and counseling. J Consult Clin Psychol 59:715–723, 1991

Foa EB, Davidson JRT, Frances A: The expert consensus guideline series: treatment of posttraumatic stress disorder. J Clin Psychiatry 60 (suppl 16):2–76, 1999

Foreman SA, Marmar CR: Therapist actions that address initially poor therapeutic alliance in psychotherapy. Am J Psychiatry 142:922–926, 1985

Frances A, Pincus HA, Widiger TA, et al: DSM-IV: work in progress. Am J Psychiatry 147:1439–1448, 1990

Frank J, Frank J: Persuasion and Healing: A Comparison Study of Psychotherapy, 3rd Edition. Baltimore, MD, Johns Hopkins University Press, 1991

Freud S: Fragment of an analysis of a case of hysteria (1905a), in The Standard Edition of the Complete Psychological Works of Sigmund Freud, Vol 7. Edited by Strachey J. London, Hogarth Press, 1953, pp 7–122

Freud S: Three essays on sexuality (1905b), in The Standard Edition of the Complete Psychological Works of Sigmund Freud, Vol 7. Edited by Strachey J. London, Hogarth Press, 1953, pp 135–243

Freud S: The dynamics of transference (1912), in The Standard Edition of the Complete Psychological Works of Sigmund Freud, Vol 12. Edited by Strachey J. London, Hogarth Press, 1958, pp 99–108

Freud S: Lines of advance in psycho-analytic therapy (1919), in The Standard Edition of the Complete Psychological Works of Sigmund Freud, Vol 17. Edited by Strachey J. London, Hogarth Press, 1964, pp 157–168

Freud S: The ego and the id (1923), in The Standard Edition of the Complete Psychological Works of Sigmund Freud, Vol 19. Edited by Strachey J. London, Hogarth Press, 1961, pp 12–66

Freud S: Inhibitions, symptoms and anxiety (1926), in The Standard Edition of the Complete Psychological Works of Sigmund Freud, Vol 20. Edited by Strachey J. London, Hogarth Press, 1959, pp 77–181

Friedman AS: Interaction of drug therapy with marital therapy in depressed patients. Arch Gen Psychiatry 32:619–637, 1975

Friedman RS, Lister P: The current status of psychodynamic formulation. Psychiatry 50:126–141, 1987

Gaston L: The concept of the alliance and its role in psychotherapy: theoretical and empirical considerations. Psychotherapy 27:143–153, 1990

Gaston L: Reliability and criterion-related validity of the California Psychotherapy Alliance Scale-Patient Version. Psychological Assessment 3:68–74, 1991

Gaston L, Marmar CR, Thompson LW, et al: Relation of patient pretreatment characteristics to the therapeutic alliance in diverse psychotherapies. J Consult Clin Psychol 56:483–489, 1988

Gill M: Analysis of the transference. J Am Psychoanal Assoc 27:263–288, 1979

Gill M: The Analysis of Transference, Vol 1. New York, International Universities Press, 1982

Gill M, Muslin H: Early interpretation of transference. J Am Psychoanal Assoc 24:779–798, 1976

Glick ID, Clarkin JF, Spencer JH, et al: A controlled evaluation of in-patient family intervention: preliminary results of the six-month follow-up. Arch Gen Psychiatry 42:882–886, 1985

Glover E: The therapeutic effect of inexact interpretation: a contribution to the theory of suggestion. International Journal of Psychoanalysis 12:397–411, 1931

Goldfried MR, Davison GC: Clinical Behavior Therapy. New York, Wiley, 1994

Goldfried MR, Raue PJ, Castonguay LG: The therapeutic focus in significant sessions of master therapists: a comparison of cognitive-behavioral and psychodynamic-interpersonal interventions. J Consult Clin Psychol 66:803–810, 1998

Goldhammer PM: Psychotherapy and pharmacotherapy: the challenge of integration. Can J Psychiatry 28:173–177, 1983

Goldman W, McCulloch J, Cuffel B, et al: Outpatient utilization patterns of integrated and split psychotherapy and pharmacotherapy for depression. Psychiatr Serv 49: 477–482, 1998

Gomes-Schwartz B: Effective ingredients in psychotherapy: prediction of outcome from process variables. J Consult Clin Psychol 46:1023–1035, 1978

Goodwin FK, Jamison KR: Manic-Depressive Illness. New York, Oxford University Press, 1990

Greenberg J, Mitchell S: Object Relations in Psychoanalytic Theory. Cambridge, MA, Harvard University Press, 1983

Greenberg LS, Rice LN, Elliott R: Facilitating Emotional Change: The Moment-By-Moment Process. New York, Guilford, 1993

Greenson RR: The Technique and Practice of Psychoanalysis, Vol 1. Madison, CT, International Universities Press, 1967

Greenson RR: The real relationship between the patient and the psychoanalyst, in The Unconscious Today. Edited by Kanzer M. New York, International Universities Press, 1971, pp 213–232

Greist JH: Treatment of obsessive-compulsiveness disorder: psychotherapies, drugs, and other somatic treatments. J Clin Psychiatry 51:44–50, 1990

Gunderson JG, Frank AF, Katz HM, et al: Effects of psychotherapy in schizophrenia, II: comparative outcome of two forms of treatment. Schizophr Bull 10:564–598, 1984

Hartley DE: Research on the therapeutic alliance in psychotherapy, in Psychiatry Update: American Psychiatric Association Annual Review, Vol 4. Edited by Hales RE, Frances AJ. Washington, DC, American Psychiatric Press, 1985, pp 532–549

Hartley D, Strupp H: The therapeutic alliance: its relationship to outcome in brief psychotherapy, in Empirical Studies of Psychoanalytic Theories. Edited by Masling J. Hillsdale, NJ, Lawrence Erlbaum, 1983, pp 1–37

Hartmann H: Ego Psychology and the Problem of Adaptation (1939). Translated by Rapaport D. New York, International Universities Press, 1958

Hartmann H, Kris E, Loewenstein R: Comments on the formation of psychic structure, in The Psychoanalytic Study of the Child, Vol 17. New York, International Universities Press, 1946, pp 42–81

Hatcher RL, Barends AW: Patients' view of the alliance in psychotherapy: exploratory factor analysis of three alliance measures. J Consult Clin Psychol 64:1326–1336, 1996

Hellerstein DJ, Rosenthal RN, Pinsker H, et al: A randomized prospective study comparing supportive and dynamic therapies. Outcome and alliance. J Psychother Pract Res 7:261–271, 1998

Henry WP, Schacht TE, Strupp HH: Structural analysis of social behavior: application to a study of interpersonal process in differential psychotherapeutic outcome. J Consult Clin Psychol 44:27–31, 1986

Henry WP, Schacht TE, Strupp HH: Patient and therapist introject, interpersonal process, and differential psychotherapy outcome. J Consult Clin Psychol 58:768–774, 1990

Henry WP, Strupp HH, Butler SF, et al: Effects of training in time-limited dynamic psychotherapy: changes in therapist behavior. J Consult Clin Psychol 61:434–440, 1993

Hoehn-Saric R: Emotional arousal, attitude change and psychotherapy, in Effective Ingredients of Successful Psychotherapy. Edited by Frank JD, Hoehn-Saric R, Imber SD, et al. New York, Brunner/Mazel, 1978, pp 73–106

Hogarty GE, Kornblith SJ, Greenwald D, et al: Three-year trials of personal therapy among schizophrenic patients living with or independent of family, I: description of study and effects on relapse rates. Am J Psychiatry 154:1504–1513, 1997

Hohagen F, Winkelmann G, Rasche-Rauchle H, et al: Combination of behaviour therapy with fluvoxamine in comparison with behavior therapy and placebo. Results of a multicentre study. Br J Psychiatry 173:71–78, 1998

Holmes SJ, Robins LN: The influence of childhood disciplinary experience on the development of alcoholism and depression. J Child Psychol Psychiatry 28:399–414, 1987

Holmes SJ, Robins LN: The role of parental disciplinary practices in the development of depression and alcoholism. Psychiatry 51:24–36, 1988

Hope DA, Heimberg RG: Social phobia and social anxiety, in Clinical Handbook of Psychological Disorders. Edited by Barlow DH. New York, Guilford, 1993, pp 99–136

Horowitz LM, Rosenberg SE, Bartholomew K: Interpersonal problems, attachment styles, and outcome in brief dynamic psychotherapy. J Consult Clin Psychol 61:549–560, 1993

Horowitz M, Marmar C: The therapeutic alliance with difficult patients, in Psychiatry Update: American Psychiatric Association Annual Review, Vol 4. Edited by Hales RE, Frances AJ. Washington, DC, American Psychiatric Press, 1985, pp 573–585

Horvath AO, Greenberg LS: Development and validation of the Working Alliance Inventory. Journal of Counseling Psychology 36:223–233, 1989

Horvath AO, Greenberg LS: The Working Alliance. New York, Wiley, 1994

Horvath AO, Symonds BD: Relation between working alliance and outcome in psychotherapy: a meta-analysis. Journal of Counseling Psychology 38:139–149, 1991

Howard K, Kopta SM, Krause MS, et al: The dose-effect relationship in psychotherapy. Am Psychol 41:159–164, 1986

Imber SD, Pilkonis PA, Sotsky SM, et al: Mode-specific effects among three treatments for depression. J Consult Clin Psychol 58:352–359, 1990

Jacobson E: The Self and the Object World. New York, International Universities Press, 1964

Jamison KR: Manic-depressive illness: the overlooked need for psychotherapy, in Integrating Pharmacotherapy and Psychotherapy. Edited by Beitman BD, Klerman GL. Washington, DC, American Psychiatric Press, 1991, pp 409–420

Jarrett RB: Comparing and combining short-term psychotherapy and pharmacotherapy for depression, in Handbook of Depression. Edited by Beckham EE, Leber WR. New York, Guilford, 1995, pp 435–464

Jones E: The Life and Work of Sigmund Freud, Vol 2. New York, Basic Books, 1955

Keller MB, Lavori PW, Mueller TI: Time to recovery, chronicity, and levels of psychopathology in major depression. Arch Gen Psychiatry 49:809–816, 1992

Keller MB, McCullough JP, Klein DN, et al: A comparison of nefazodone, the cognitive behavioral-analysis system of psychotherapy, and their combination for the treatment of chronic depression. N Engl J Med 342:1462–1470, 2000

Kessler RC, McGonagle KA, Zhao S, et al: Lifetime and 12-month prevalence of DSM-III-R psychiatric disorders in the United States. Arch Gen Psychiatry 51:8–19, 1994

Klerman GL: Ideological conflicts in integrating pharmacotherapy and psychotherapy, in Integrating Pharmacotherapy and Psychotherapy. Edited by Beitman BD, Klerman GL. Washington, DC, American Psychiatric Press, 1991, pp 3–19

Klerman GL, Weissman MM, Rounsaville BJ, et al: Interpersonal Psychotherapy of Depression. New York, Basic Books, 1984

Koenigsberg HW: Borderline personality disorder, in Integrating Pharmacotherapy and Psychotherapy. Edited by Beitman BD, Klerman GL. Washington, DC, American Psychiatric Press, 1991, pp 271–290

Kohlenberg BS, Yeater EA, Kohlenberg RJ: Functional analytic psychotherapy, the therapeutic alliance, and brief psychotherapy, in The Therapeutic Alliance in Brief Psychotherapy. Edited by Safran JD, Muran JC. Washington, DC, American Psychological Association Books, 1998, pp 63–93

Kohlenberg RJ, Tsai M: Functional Analytic Psychotherapy: Creating Intense and Curative Therapeutic Relationships. New York, Plenum, 1991

Kohut H: The Analysis of the Self. New York, International Universities Press, 1971

Kohut H: The Restoration of the Self. New York, International Universities Press, 1977

Kovacs M, Beck AT: Maladaptive cognitive structures in depression. Am J Psychiatry 135:525–533, 1978

Lafferty P, Beutler LE, Crago M: Differences between more or less effective psychotherapists: a study of select therapist variables. J Consult Clin Psychol 57:76–80, 1989

Laikin M, Winston A, McCullough L: Intensive short-term dynamic psychotherapy, in Handbook of Short-Term Dynamic Psychotherapy. Edited by Crits-Christoph P, Barber JP. New York, Basic Books, 1991, pp 80–109

Lambert MJ: Some implications of psychotherapy outcome research for eclectic psychotherapy. International Journal of Eclectic Psychotherapy 16:16–45, 1986

Lambert MJ: The individual therapist's contribution to psychotherapy process and outcome. Clin Psychol Rev 9:469–485, 1989

Lambert MJ, Bergin AE: The effectiveness of psychotherapy, in Handbook of Psychotherapy and Behavior Change. Edited by Bergin AE, Garfield SL. New York, Wiley, 1994, pp 143–189

Langs R: The Listening Process. New York, Jason Aronson, 1978

Lavori PW, Keller MB, Mueller TI, et al: Recurrence after recovery in unipolar MDD: an observational follow-up study of clinical predictors and somatic treatment as a mediating factor. International Journal of Methods in Psychiatric Research 4: 211–229, 1994

Levenson E: The Ambiguity of Change: An Inquiry Into the Nature of Psychoanalytic Reality. New York, Basic Books, 1983

Lewis J: To Be a Therapist: The Teaching and Learning. New York, Brunner/Mazel, 1978

Lindemann E: Symptomatology and management of acute grief. Am J Psychiatry 101: 141–148, 1944

Luborsky L: Helping alliances in psychotherapy, in Successful Psychotherapy. Edited by Claghorn JL. New York, Brunner/Mazel, 1976, pp 92–116

Luborsky L: Measuring a pervasive psychic structure in psychotherapy: the core conflictual relationship theme, in Communicative Structures and Psychic Structures. Edited by Freedman N, Grand S. New York, Plenum, 1977, pp 367–395

Luborsky L: Principles of Psychoanalytic Psychotherapy: A Manual for Supportive-Expressive Treatment. New York, Basic Books, 1984

Luborsky L, Crits-Christoph P: Understanding Transference: The CCRT Method. New York, Basic Books, 1990

Luborsky L, Crits-Christoph P, Alexander L, et al: Two helping alliance methods for predicting outcomes of psychotherapy: a counting sign vs a global rating method. J Nerv Ment Dis 171:480–492, 1983

Luborsky L, Crits-Christoph P, McLellan AT, et al: Do therapists vary much in their success? Findings from four outcome studies. Am J Orthopsychiatry 56:501–512, 1986

Luborsky L, Diguer L, Luborsky E, et al: The efficacy of dynamic psychotherapies: is it true that "everyone has won and all must have prizes"? in Psychodynamic Treatment Research. Edited by Miller NE, Luborsky L, Barber JP, et al. New York, Basic Books, 1993, pp 497–516

Luborsky L, Singer B, Luborsky E: Comparative studies of psychotherapy: is it true that "everybody has won and all must have prizes"? Arch Gen Psychiatry 32: 995–1008, 1975

MacKenzie KR: The alliance in time-limited group psychotherapy, in The Therapeutic Alliance in Brief Psychotherapy. Edited by Safran JD, Muran JC. Washington, DC, American Psychological Association Books, 1998, pp 193–216

Mahler MS: On Human Symbiosis and the Vicissitudes of Individuation. New York, International Universities Press, 1968

Mahler MS, Pine F, Bergman A: The Psychological Birth of the Human Infant. New York, Basic Books, 1975

Mahoney MJ: Cognition and Behavior Modification. Cambridge, MA, Ballinger, 1974

Malan DH: A Study of Brief Psychotherapy. New York, Plenum, 1963

Malan DH: The Frontier of Brief Psychotherapy. New York, Plenum, 1976

Malan DH: Individual Psychotherapy and the Science of Psychodynamics. London, Butterworth, 1979

Mann J: Time-Limited Psychotherapy. Cambridge, MA, Harvard University Press, 1973

Mann J: Time-limited psychotherapy, in Short-Term Dynamic Psychotherapy. Edited by Crits-Christoph P, Barber JP. New York, Basic Books, 1991, pp 17–43

Marks I: Behavioural and drug treatments of phobic and obsessive-compulsive disorders. Psychother Psychosom 46:35–44, 1986

Marmar CR, Horowitz MJ, Weiss DS, et al: Development of the therapeutic rating system, in The Psychotherapeutic Process: A Research Handbook. Edited by Greenberg LS, Pinsof WM. New York, Guilford, 1986, pp 367–390

Marmar CR, Weiss DS, Gaston L: Toward the validation of the California Therapeutic Alliance Rating System. Psychological Assessment 1:46–52, 1989

Marziali E: Prediction of outcome of brief psychotherapy from therapist interpretive interventions. Arch Gen Psychiatry 41:301–305, 1984

Mattick RP, Peters L: Treatment of severe social phobia: effects of guided exposure with and without cognitive restructuring. J Consult Clin Psychol 56:251–260, 1988

Mattick RP, Peters L, Clark JC: Exposure and cognitive restructuring for severe social phobia: a controlled study. Behavior Therapy 20:3–23, 1989

McCullough L, Winston A, Farber BA, et al: The relationship of patient-therapist interaction to outcome in brief psychotherapy. Psychotherapy 28:525–533, 1991

McLellan AT, Woody G, Luborsky L, et al: Increased effectiveness of substance abuse treatment. A prospective study of patient-treatment "matching." J Nerv Ment Dis 171:597–605, 1983

Meichenbaum DH: Cognitive Behavior Modification. New York, Plenum, 1977

Meichenbaum DH, Goodman J: Training impulsive children to talk to themselves. J Abnorm Psychol 77:127–132, 1971

Mendelson GA, Geller MH: Similarity, missed sessions, and early termination. Journal of Counseling Psychology 14:210–215, 1967

Menninger K: Theory of Psychoanalytic Technique. London, Imago, 1958

Miklowitz DJ: Psychotherapy in combination with drug treatment for bipolar disorder. J Clin Psychopharmacology 16 (suppl 1):565–665, 1996

Mitchell S: Relational Concepts in Psychoanalysis: An Integration. Cambridge, MA, Harvard University Press, 1988

Moore BE, Fine BD: Psychoanalytic Terms and Concepts. Binghamton, NY, Vail-Ballou, 1990, pp 44–45

Moras K, Strupp H: Pretherapy interpersonal relations, patients' alliance, and outcome in brief therapy. Arch Gen Psychiatry 39:405–409, 1982

Muran JC, Ventur E: The operant self. The Behavior Therapist 18:91–94, 1995

Muran JC, Segal ZV, Samstag LW, et al: Patient pretreatment interpersonal problems and the therapeutic alliance. J Consult Clin Psychol 62:185–190, 1994

Muran JC, Samstag LW, Jilton R, et al: Development of a suboutcome strategy to measure interpersonal process in psychotherapy from an observer perspective. J Clin Psychol 53:405–420, 1997

Muskin PR: The combined use of psychotherapy and pharmacotherapy in the medical setting. Psychiatr Clin North Am 13:341–53, 1990

Neisser U: Cognitive Psychology. New York, Appleton-Century-Crofts, 1967

Nelson JC, Bowers MB Jr: Delusional unipolar depression: description and drug response. Arch Gen Psychiatry 35:1321–1328, 1978

Novalis PN, Rojcewicz SJ, Peele R: Clinical Manual of Supportive Psychotherapy. Washington, DC, American Psychiatric Press, 1993

Nunberg H: The synthetic function of the ego. International Journal of Psychoanalysis 12:123–140, 1931

Orford J: The rules of interpersonal complementarity: does hostility beget hostility and dominance, submission? Psychological Review 93:365–377, 1986

Orlinsky DE, Howard KI: Gender and psychotherapeutic outcome, in Woman and Psychotherapy. Edited by Brodsky AM, Hare-Mustin RT. New York, Guilford, 1980, pp 3–34

Pardes H, Papernik D, Winston A: Field differentiation in inpatient psychotherapy. Arch Gen Psychiatry 31:311–315, 1974

Parloff MB: Goals in psychotherapy: mediating and ultimate, in Goals of Psychotherapy. Edited by Mahrer AR. New York, Appleton-Century-Crofts, 1967, pp 5–19

Parloff MB, Waskow IE, Wolfe BE: Research on therapist variables in relation to process and outcome, in Handbook of Psychotherapy and Behavior Change. Edited by Garfield SL, Bergin AE. New York, Wiley, 1978, pp 233–282

Perry JC, Banon E, Ianni F: Effectiveness of psychotherapy for personality disorders. Am J Psychiatry 156:1312–1321, 1999

Perry S, Cooper AM, Michels R: The psychodynamic formulation: its purpose, structure, and clinical application. Am J Psychiatry 144:543–550, 1987

Persons JB: Cognitive Therapy in Practice: A Case Formulation Approach. New York, WW Norton, 1989

Persons JB: Case conceptualization in cognitive-behavior therapy, in Cognitive Therapy in Action: Evolving Innovative Practice. Edited by Kuchlwein KT, Rosen H. San Francisco, CA, Jossey-Bass, 1993, pp 33–53

Pinsker H: A Primer of Supportive Psychotherapy. Hillsdale, NJ, Analytic Press, 1998

Pinsker H, Rosenthal R, McCullough L: Dynamic supportive psychotherapy, in Handbook of Brief Dynamic Psychotherapies. Edited by Crits-Christoph P, Barber JP. New York, Basic Books, 1991, pp 220–247

Piper WE, Azim HFA, Joyce AS, et al: Transference interpretation, therapeutic alliance, and outcome in short-term individual psychotherapy. Arch Gen Psychiatry 48:946–953, 1991

Piper WE, Debbane EG, Bienvenu JP, et al: Relationships between the object focus of therapist interpretations and outcome in short-term individual psychotherapy. Br J Med Psychol 59:1–11, 1986

Piper WE, Joyce AS, McCallum M, et al: Interpretive and supportive forms of psychotherapy and patient personality variables. J Consult Clin Psychol 66:558–567, 1998

Pollack J, Flegenheimer W, Winston A: Brief adaptive psychotherapy, in Handbook of Short-Term Dynamic Psychotherapy. Edited by Crits-Christoph P, Barber JP. New York, Basic Books, 1991, pp 199–219

Post RM: Transduction of psychosocial stress into the neurobiology of recurrent affective disorder. Am J Psychiatry 149:999–1010, 1992

Rachman SJ, Wilson GT: The Effects of Psychological Therapy, 2nd Edition. New York, Pergamon, 1980

Rank O: The Trauma of Birth (1929). New York, Harper & Row, 1973

Regier DA, Farmer ME, Rae DS, et al: Co-morbidity of mental disorders with alcohol and other drug abuse: results from the Epidemiologic Catchment Area (ECA) Study. JAMA 264:2511–2518, 1990

Reich W: Character Analysis (1933), 3rd Edition. Translated by Wolfe TP. New York, Orgone Institute Press, 1949

Reynolds CF, Frank E, Perel JM, et al: Combined pharmacotherapy and psychotherapy in the acute and continuation treatment of elderly patients with recurrent major depression: a preliminary report. Am J Psychiatry 149:1687–1692, 1992

Reynolds CF, Miller MD, Pasternak RE, et al: Treatment of bereavement-related major depressive episodes in later life: a controlled study of acute and continuation treatment with nortriptyline and interpersonal psychotherapy. Am J Psychiatry 156:202–208, 1999

Robinson LA, Berman JS, Neimeyer RA: Psychotherapy for the treatment of depression: a comprehensive review of controlled outcome research. Psychol Bull 100: 30–49, 1990

Rockland LH: Supportive Therapy: A Psychodynamic Approach. New York, Basic Books, 1989

Rosenthal RN, Muran JC, Hellerstein DJ, et al: Interpersonal change in supportive psychotherapy. J Psychother Pract Res 8:55–63, 1999

Rosenzweig S: Some implicit common factors in diverse methods of psychotherapy. Am J Orthopsychiatry 6:412–415, 1936

Roth D, Bielski R, Jones M, et al: A comparison of self-control therapy and combined self-control therapy and antidepressant medication in the treatment of depression. Behavior Therapy 13:133–144, 1982

Rounsaville BJ, Klerman GL, Weissman MM: Do psychotherapy and pharmacotherapy for depression conflict? Empirical evidence from a clinical trial. Arch Gen Psychiatry 38:24–29, 1981

Ryle A: The focus in brief interpretive psychotherapy: dilemmas, traps and snags as target problems. Br J Psychiatry 134:46–54, 1979

Sabin JE: Short-term group psychotherapy: historical antecedent, in Forms of Brief Therapy. Edited by Budman SH. New York, Guilford, 1981, pp 271–282

Safran JD, Muran JC: The Therapeutic Alliance in Brief Psychotherapy. Washington, DC, American Psychological Association Books, 1998

Safran JD, Muran JC: Negotiating the Therapeutic Alliance: A Relational Treatment Guide. New York, Guilford, 2000

Safran JD, Segal ZV: Interpersonal Process in Cognitive Therapy. New York, Basic Books, 1990

Safran JD, Crocker P, McMain S, et al: The Therapeutic alliance rupture as a therapy event for empirical investigation. Psychotherapy: Theory, Research, and Practice 27:154–165, 1990

Safran JD, Muran JC, Samstag LW: Resolving therapeutic alliance ruptures: a task analytic investigation, in The Working Alliance: Theory, Research and Practice. Edited by Horvath AO, Greenberg LS. New York, Wiley, 1994, pp 225–255

Samstag LW, Batchelder ST, Muran JC, et al: Early identification of treatment failures in short-term psychotherapy. An assessment of therapeutic alliance and interpersonal behavior. J Psychother Pract Res 7:126–143, 1998

Segal ZV, Shaw BF: Cognitive therapy, in The American Psychiatric Press Review of Psychiatry, Vol 15. Edited by Dickstein LJ, Riba MB, Oldham JM. Washington, DC, American Psychiatric Press, 1996, pp 69–90

Sensky T, Turkington D, Kingdon D, et al: A randomized controlled trial of cognitive-behavioral therapy for persistent symptoms in schizophrenia resistant to medication. Arch Gen Psychiatry 57:163–172, 2000

Shapiro DA: Comparative creditability of treatment rationales: three tests of expectancy theory. Br J Clin Psychol 21:111–122, 1981

Shapiro DA, Barkham M, Rees A, et al: Effects of treatment duration and severity of depression on the effectiveness of cognitive-behavioral and psychodynamic-interpersonal psychotherapy. J Consult Clin Psychol 62:522–534, 1994

Shapiro DA, Rees A, Barkham M, et al: Effects of treatment duration and severity of depression on the maintenance of gains after cognitive-behavioral and psychodynamic-interpersonal psychotherapy. J Consult Clin Psychol 63:378–387, 1995

Shea MT, Elkin I, Hirschfeld RMA: Psychotherapeutic treatment of depression, in Review of Psychiatry, Vol 7. Edited by Francis A, Hales RE. Washington, DC, American Psychiatric Press, 1988, pp 235–255

Sifneos PE: Short-Term Psychotherapy and Emotional Crisis. Cambridge, MA, Harvard University Press, 1972

Sifneos PE: Short-Term Dynamic Psychotherapy: Evaluation and Technique. New York, Plenum, 1979

Singer E: The interpersonal approach to psychoanalysis, in Current Theories of Psychoanalysis. Edited by Langs R. Madison, CT, International Universities Press, 1998, pp 73–101

Smith M, Glass G, Miller T: The Benefits of Psychotherapy. Baltimore, MD, Johns Hopkins University Press, 1980

Sotsky SM, Glass DR, Shea MT, et al: Patient predictors of response to psychotherapy and pharmacotherapy: findings in the NIMH Treatment of Depression Collaborative Research Program. Am J Psychiatry 148:997–1008, 1991

Spitz R: The First Year of Life. New York, International Universities Press, 1965

Stern DN: The Interpersonal World of the Infant: A View From Psychoanalysis and Developmental Psychology. New York, Basic Books, 1985

Stern DN, Sander LW, Nahum JP, et al: Non-interpretive mechanisms in psychoanalytic therapy. The 'something more' than interpretation. The Process of Change Study Group. Int J Psychoanal 79(Pt 5):903–921, 1998

Stewart RL: Psychoanalysis and psychoanalytic psychotherapy, in Comprehensive Textbook of Psychiatry, 4th Edition. Edited by Kaplan HI, Sadock BJ. Baltimore, MD, Williams & Wilkins, 1985, pp 1331–1365

Strupp HH: The Vanderbilt Psychotherapy Studies: synopsis. J Consult Clin Psychol 61:431–433, 1993

Strupp HH: The psychotherapist's skills revisited. Clinical Psychology: Science and Practice 2:70–74, 1995

Strupp HH, Binder JL: Psychotherapy in a New Key: A Guide to Time-Limited Psychotherapy. New York, Basic Books, 1984

Stiles WB, Agnew-Davies R, Hardy GE, et al: Relations of the alliance with psychotherapy outcome: findings in the Second Sheffield Psychotherapy Project. J Consult Clin Psychol 66:791–802, 1998

Sullivan HS: Conception of Modern Psychiatry. New York, WW Norton, 1953

Sullivan M, Verhulst J, Russo J, et al: Psychotherapy vs pharmacotherapy: are psychiatrists polarized? A survey of academic and clinical faculty. Am J Psychotherapy 47:411–423, 1993

Talley PF, Strupp HH, Morey LC: Matchmaking in psychotherapy: patient-therapist dimensions and their impact on outcome. J Consult Clin Psychol 58:182–188, 1990

Tarachow S: An Introduction to Psychotherapy. New York, International Universities Press, 1963

Thase ME: Integrating psychotherapy and pharmacotherapy for treatment of major depressive disorder. Current status and future considerations. J Psychother Pract Res 6:300–306, 1997

Thase ME, Greenhouse JB, Frank E, et al: Treatment of major depression with psychotherapy or psychotherapy-pharmacotherapy combinations. Arch Gen Psychiatry 54:1009–1015, 1997

Tolpin M: On the beginnings of a cohesive self: an application of the concept of transmuting internalization to the study of the transitional object and signal anxiety, in The Psychoanalytic Study of the Child, Vol 26. New York, Quadrangle Books, 1972, pp 316–352

Tomkins SS: Affect, Imagery, and Consciousness, Vol 1: Positive Affects. New York, Springer, 1962

Tomkins SS: Affect, Imagery, and Consciousness, Vol 2: Negative Affects. New York, Springer, 1963

Tomkins SS: Affect, Imagery, and Consciousness, Vol 4: Cognition. New York, Springer, 1992

Tompkins MA: Cognitive-behavioral case formulation: the case of Jim. Journal of Psychotherapy Integration 6:97–105, 1996

Tuma AH, May PRA, Yale C, et al: Therapist characteristics and the outcome of treatment in schizophrenia. Arch Gen Psychiatry 34:81–85, 1978

Twillman RK, Manetto C: Concurrent psychotherapy and pharmacotherapy in the treatment of depression and anxiety in cancer patients. Psychooncology 7:285–290, 1998

Vaillant GE: Adaptation to Life. Boston, MA, Little, Brown, 1977

Vaillant GE (ed): Empirical Studies of Ego Mechanisms of Defense. Washington, DC, American Psychiatric Press, 1986

Vaughan SC, Roose SP, Marshall RD, et al: Affective disorders and psychodynamic treatment. Paper presented at the annual meeting of the American Psychiatric Association, San Diego, CA, May 1997

Wallace ER: Dynamic Psychiatry in Theory and Practice. Philadelphia, PA, Lea & Febiger, 1983, pp 345–346

Wallerstein RS: The Psychotherapy Research Project of the Menninger Foundation: an overview. J Consult Clin Psychol 57:195–205, 1989

Walsh BT, Wilson GT, Terence G, et al: Medication and psychotherapy in the treatment of bulimia nervosa. Am J Psychiatry 154:523–531, 1997

Walter B: Theme and Variations. New York, Knopf, 1946

Weiss J, Sampson H, the Mount Zion Psychotherapy Research Group: The Psychoanalytic Process: Theory, Clinical Observations, and Empirical Research. New York, Guilford, 1986

Weissman MM: The psychological treatment of depression. Evidence for the efficacy of psychotherapy alone, in comparison with, and in combination with pharmacotherapy. Arch Gen Psychiatry 36:1261–1269, 1979

Weissman MM, Kasl SV, Klerman GL: Follow-up of depressed women after maintenance treatment. Am J Psychiatry 133:757–760, 1976

Weissman MM, Klerman GL, Prusoff BA, et al: Depressed outpatients: results one year after treatment with drugs and/or interpersonal psychotherapy. Arch Gen Psychiatry 38:51–55, 1981

Weissman MM, Markowitz JC, Klerman GL: Comprehensive Guide to Interpersonal Psychotherapy. New York, Basic Books, 2000

Werman DS: The Practice of Supportive Psychotherapy. New York, Brunner/Mazel, 1984

Westerman MA, Foote JP, Winston A: Change in coordination across phases of psychotherapy and outcome: two mechanisms for the role played by patients' contribution to the alliance. J Consult Clin Psychol 24:190–195, 1995

Whitehorn JC, Betz BJ: Further studies of the doctor as a crucial variable in the outcome of treatment with schizophrenic patients. Am J Psychiatry 117:215–223, 1960

Wierzbicki M, Pekarik G: A meta-analysis of psychotherapy drop-out. Professional Psychology: Research and Practice 24:190–195, 1993

Wiggins JS: Circumplex models of interpersonal behavior in clinical psychology, in Handbook of Research Methods in Clinical Psychology. Edited by Kendell C, Butcher JN. New York, Wiley, 1982, pp 183–221

Wilson PH: Combined pharmacological and behavioural treatment of depression. Behav Res Ther 20:173–184, 1982

Winnicott DW: The Maturational Process and the Facilitating Environment: Studies in the Theory of Emotional Development. London, Hogarth Press, 1965

Winston A, Muran JC: Common factors in the time-limited psychotherapies, in The American Psychiatric Press Review of Psychiatry, Vol 15. Edited by Dickstein LJ, Riba MB, Oldham JM. Washington, DC, American Psychiatric Press, 1996, pp 43–68

Winston A, Pinsker H, McCullough L: A review of supportive psychotherapy. Hospital and Community Psychiatry 37:1105–1114, 1986

Winston A, Pollack J, McCullough L, et al: Brief dynamic psychotherapy of personality disorders. J Nerv Ment Dis 179:188–193, 1991

Winston A, Laikin M, Pollack J: Short-term psychotherapy of personality disorders. Am J Psychiatry 151:190–194, 1994a

Winston A, Muran JC, Samstag LW: Pretreatment predictors of the therapeutic alliance. Paper presented at the annual meeting of the Society for Psychotherapy Research, York, England, June 1994b

Winston A, Rosenthal RN, Muran JC: Supportive psychotherapy, in Handbook of Personality Disorders. Edited by Livesley WJ. New York, Guilford, 2001, pp 344–358

Winston B, Winston A, Samstag LW, et al: Patient defense/therapist interventions. Psychotherapy 31:478–491, 1994

Wolf ES: Empathy and countertransference, in The Future of Psychoanalysis. Edited by Goldberg A. New York, International Universities Press, 1983, pp 309–326

Young JE: Cognitive Therapy for Personality Disorders: A Schema-Focused Approach. Sarasota, FL, Professional Resource Exchange, 1990

Zetzel E: Current concepts of transference. International Journal of Psychoanalysis 37:369–375, 1956

Zetzel E: The analytic situation, in Psychoanalysis in America. New York, International Universities Press, 1966, pp 86–106

Index

Page numbers printed in **boldface** type refer to tables and figures.